STRESSMANSHIP

D0234621

THE AUTHOR

Dr Audrey Livingston Booth trained at Guy's Hospital before taking a certificate in Tropical Medicine at the School of Tropical Diseases. After marrying and becoming a mother, she studied Froebel teaching, health education, sociology and psychology and finally took a doctorate in neuro-psychology. She has had a varied career and has, amongst other things, been Froebel Institute Senior Lecturer in health education and is a Lecturer of the Institute of Education, London University. She is now Director of the Stress Foundation.

THE STRESS FOUNDATION

The Stress Foundation was founded in 1981. Because of the increase in coronary heart disease and pyschosomatic and stress-related illnesses, its Board of Trustees believed that such a foundation was necessary to educate and advise both industry and the public about the effects of stress. It is a charitable institution and has an interdisciplinary Scientific Council.

STRESSMANSHIP

by

Dr Audrey Livingston Booth

Director
of
THE STRESS FOUNDATION

Severn House Publishers

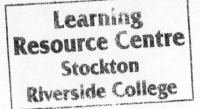

Learning
Resource Centre
Stockton
Riverside College

616.8

This first world edition published in 1985 by
SEVERN HOUSE PUBLISHERS LTD of
40–42 William IV Street, London WC2N 4DF

Reprinted 1986, 1988

Copyright © Audrey Livingston Booth, 1985

British Library Cataloguing in Publication Data
Livingston Booth, Audrey
Stressmanship
1. Stress (Psychology)   2. Stress (Physiology)
I. Title
616.8   BF575.S75
ISBN 0–7278–2054–0
ISBN 0–7278–2088–5 Pbk

All rights reserved. No part of this publication may be
reproduced, stored in a retrieval system, rebound or
transmitted in any form or by any means, electronic,
mechanical, photocopying, recording or otherwise, without
the prior permission of Severn House Publishers Limited.

Typeset by Inforum Ltd, Portsmouth
Printed and bound in Great Britain at
the University Printing House, Oxford

Acknowledgements

All authors, and I am no exception, owe so much to previous writers and researchers whose work, often unwittingly perhaps, influences their thinking, feeling and perceptions of a subject – those are the unknown, whom I thank.

The known influences are many. From the early days I owe a great deal to Professor Mackintosh who was Professor of Public Health, to John Burton and Winifred Warden who led me into Health Education and to Dorothy Gardner who did the same for Psychology.

Among later influences were Professor Bernstein and Michael Young for Sociology, but above all there was Dr Mel Marshak who guided me through Neurology and Child Development for four years of inspirational tutoring which so widened my horizons and my thinking. To her I owe a very special debt of gratitude.

Coming to the present time, I do want to record my thanks for the unfailing support I have recieved from the Management of the Stress Foundation, Sir Monty Finniston, President, Professor Linford Rees, Vice-President, and Mr Walter Goldsmith, Chairman, and the members of the Board of Trustees and the Scientific Advisory Council. To them goes a very special debt of gratitude for their unstinting help, advice and encouragement. However, any expressions of opinion or conclusions drawn from research quoted in the book are my own, and do not necessarily represent the views of the Foundation.

My very warm and heartfelt thanks go to my husband Dick Livingston Booth for his patient translation of 'gobble-de-gook' into the Queen's English, and to Julian Mannering of Severn House for his unfailing encouragement.

Contents

PART III

Stress-induced
illnesses and
professional help

Stress and its causes

Today, most people would say that there is stress in their lives – indeed far too many would claim to be under real strain. The stress that most of us know can be felt in the draining emotional tiredness born of all those little daily irritations and frustrations, the niggles and the petty rows, the flare-ups and the back-biting, each in themselves a symptom of stress. Stress tiredness is a kind of deadness or numb feeling which so often leads to the thought 'I daren't stop and sit down because if I do I'll never get going again'. This is quite different from the pleasantly relaxed, warm tiredness we experience after a job well done as we sink back into a comfortable chair with a contented sigh.

We feel stress in the headache that starts at the back of the neck and creeps over the top of the head, or settles in a band of pressure all round the head. We see it in our displacement activities of doing anything other than the thing we should be getting on with. We see it in the nail-biting, hair-twirling, child; in the hand of the driver beating a tattoo on the steering wheel while stuck in a traffic jam; in the fiery response to an innocent question; in the over-hearty laugh, the doubling of our cigarette consumption, and the craving for the stimulus of hot spicy food, exotic drinks and sexual excitement. *The signs of stress*

In the more advanced stages of stress we hate ourselves for swearing at our children, bawling out that nice new junior for a trivial mistake, and kicking the cat for no better reason than we feel as taut as an over-tuned violin string. Sometimes we wonder that it does not snap – or perhaps we *The signs of real strain*

9

secretly fear that one day it will. We lie awake at night reliving the day's events from 1 am to 3 am, longing for sleep or for the dawn. But when daylight does come we just do not want to get up and face all those problems all over again. Yes, we certainly know what stress is.

A twentieth century illness

This pattern of being uptight, under pressure, anxious or depressed, seems to be a rapidly growing misfortune of modern Western society, an explosion lacking explanation or understanding, leaving each of us helpless and alone with a problem which we are reluctant to admit to our families or friends, and for which we see no solution. For many believe that not only is stress a major cause of illness, particularly 'heart attacks' or 'strokes', but that it cannot be recognised or prevented, and there is no treatment for it except tranquillisers which only treat the symptoms and not the cause.

To deal with stress

These beliefs are tragic for society as a whole, but particularly so for the individuals who suffer. Indeed, when a large part of the population believes that coronary heart disease, which is the most frequent killer in the United Kingdom, is brought about by something which cannot be recognised, prevented or cured, it is high time to sweep away the myths and establish the facts. For example, how many people know that we all have a mechanism in the body which deals with stress? We have. It is deep in the brain and it switches on to help us over emergencies or threats and all the challenges for which we need extra energy. How many times have you said 'I don't know how I coped with that, but somehow I had the strength to get through all right'. The strength came from our 'stress response', our answer to stress. It provides a powerhouse of energy which, when harnessed, will give you that 'get up and go' feeling essential to success. This book will tell you how to harness it.

Stress is good when harnessed

Stress itself is a good and valuable human response to challenge or change. It is an essential and useful part of a healthy life. But if it is not harnessed or controlled it can drive us to disaster as when we have been driving for too long with the accelerator hard down, the engine over-heating and the bodywork shaking to bits. Stress can be identified in ourselves and in others, and any bad effects can be prevented, or cured without drugs.

10

The book is arranged in three parts.

Part I deals with exactly what stress is, what the different stages are, whether they are good or bad and what the signs and symptoms of each stage are. It helps you to recognise each stage in yourself and in other people. It tells you why we have so much stress today, and who among us are most stressed.

Part II really gets down to the business of what to do about it. You will find a personality test to indicate the extent to which you are at risk from stress. You will find first aid tension reducers to help you through a hectic day, and long-term measures to prevent stress from knocking you down again. There are chapters which tell you how to build a balanced lifestyle; give you the low-down on food and slimming; tell you how to handle anxiety and depression and how to experience unstressed intimate relationships. The whole is intended to enable you to drive yourself hard, when necessary, without running the risk of overheating and burning out.

Part III leads you to sources of additional help if you feel you need it. It explains the roles of the general practitioner, the psychiatrist, the psychologist, and the counsellor. It discusses the help that is available in complementary medicine, from acupuncture to naturopathy, and tells you how to set about finding accredited practitioners.

Throughout the book there are quizzes to help you find your own stress scores. You should be able to reduce some immediately and others within a few weeks. Within three months you should have made considerable strides in mastering stress. Do not let it master you and drive you to despair. It can be controlled. Look around at the successful people who have done it. What they have done, you can do too.

CHAPTER 1

Stressmanship

Just as gamesmanship means far more than just knowing how to play a game, stressmanship is more than just knowing how to control stress. It covers the entire art (and it is an art) of understanding and handling stress. It is getting to grips with it so thoroughly that you not only understand it, but you know what to do about it for yourself, your colleagues, your family and your friends. In fact, it is more than that even. It is actually about staying alive, for it is no earthly good trying to make Secretary of the Year or the youngest ever Consultant or Company Chairman at the age of twenty-eight, and having a heart attack at thirty, is it?

It is also about living healthily and happily, because life itself is no fun if you are in a state of anxiety or depression and there is no one to help you over it. Stressmanship is about managing and conquering both, and also the fears, panic and phobias that can accompany high anxiety. It is about developing friendships and building up support groups both at home and at work. It is about coping with the stress of loss, in which we lose a part of ourselves, whether the loss is of a child, husband, parent or lover. It is about coping with the loss of a job through enforced early retirement, redundancy or temporary lay-off. We have, as it were, lost our place in society and we feel bitter and angry at the loss of status, and again, the loss of a part of ourselves – our 'work self'. It is about boredom – the unrelenting, dull monotony of a routine job which satisfies neither our emotions nor our intelligence. One can be literally bored to death.

A happy life

Further, it is about the development of contentment. This is the opposite of what we are taught by the striving, achieving, acquisitive society. One way to develop this is to look outside our artificially created, time controlled world

Developing contentment

13

to the natural world surrounding us. This helps to reduce stress because of the emotional satisfaction the natural world gives to us. Those who begin to take the time to look about them, to use their senses more intensely, to listen to the song of the birds, or to watch the play of sunlight on leaves, are rewarded by a growing sense of quietness and pleasure. Then we remember the joy and the wonder we once had in the world about us before we became too busy and too bogged down to notice. Yes, you can build it into your very busy schedule because if you don't, there may very well be no schedule to build it into – or no you. It really is no use being the fastest thing on two legs or the pride and joy of the typing pool, and suffering from anxiety, depression or the shakes. We have to get the balance of our health right. Once upon a time, remember, you could cope with everything. Then everything got on top of you. Why? Read the next Chapter, *Getting to grips with stress*, and you will understand and then really get to grips with life again.

Physical and emotional stress differ

We need to know the difference between physical and emotional stress. We can subject the body to a great deal of physical stress like exercise, heavy gardening, sawing logs and the like, and muscles will ache. After a hot bath, a drink, a rest and a relaxing evening (easy after physical tiredness), we are as good as new. Emotional stress is different. We become much more highly aroused and tensed up. In fact, the emotional stress for a student of facing a final examination, or for some of us even a visit to the dentist, can be as high as the very highest level of physical stress, for example, the undergoing of a major surgical operation. This is fact, proven by checking the levels of the stress chemicals found in the body during different experiences.

You can identify stress

Stress can be identified today. Stressmanship is identifying it; knowing that we have got it; knowing why we have stress today in the twentieth century. It is knowing what to do about it, and it is knowing when we need outside help and where and how to get it. It is knowing whether we need our doctor, a psychiatrist, a psychologist, psychotherapy or yoga. Take this business of knowing whether we have got it. How many of us really know if we are stressed or not? We only know that we feel rotten, miserable, down or depressed; and that it takes very little to make us burst into

14

tears, scream or go out and get drunk. We are certainly not the ball of fun, fire and enthusiasm we once were.

How many of the following phrases do you regularly use? *Is this you?*
- I feel just as tired when I wake up as I did when I went to bed.
- I just cannot face another day with that individual in the office. I wonder if I could go sick?
- (As the alarm bell rings) Oh Lord, another day.
- I used to like my job. Now I couldn't care less.
- It's no good me sitting down – I'll never get started again.
- I get so bad tempered with the children lately, and its really not like me.
- Life has become one long, boring slog these days.
- Isn't life maddening – nothing ever goes right?
- I think I need a drink before facing that.

Well, let's find out. Below are some symptoms of stress. *How much* Look at them carefully and tick every one you have. *stress do you have?*

- I have frequent headaches although my doctor says that *My mind* there is nothing wrong with me.
- I sometimes hear head noises, ringing or buzzing in the ears.
- My memory seems to have gone lately.
- I can't stop thinking about one particular thing or tune and it goes round and round in my head.
- I can't seem to settle down and get on with things I have to do: I keep putting them off.
- I can't concentrate on anything these days.
- My head often feels full of cotton wool and I can't think through it.

- My legs twitch in bed at night and I frequently have *My body* cramp.
- I often have aches or pains in the back of the neck but my doctor says that there is nothing wrong.
- My shoulders and back ache a lot at the end of the day – without having had hard physical exercise.
- I sometimes have difficulty in keeping my hands from trembling.
- I sigh often.
- I sometimes feel that I cannot get enough breath in my lungs.

15

- I sometimes feel that I am going to pass out.
- I frequently have diarrhoea. I have had tests and they say there is nothing wrong.
- Sometimes my rings get very tight and I have difficulty doing up my skirt or trousers.
- I am sometimes very gassy and burp a lot.
- Some days I frequently need to go to the loo to pass water. I'm told there is nothing the matter with me.
- I take a long time to go to sleep.
- I frequently wake up in the early hours and have difficulty in getting back to sleep.
- I get very hot at night and my heart-beat seems louder and faster.
- My heart seems to skip beats, but the doctor says it is quite healthy.

My social life
- People at work are very difficult.
- There are too many demands on me and too much change.
- I have no real friend to confide in.
- Life is nothing but work and sleep.
- I have family problems.
- I don't really know anyone.

My emotional life
- I am often very near to tears.
- I rarely laugh these days.
- I react to everything with the same feeling. There aren't any ups or downs any more.
- The least little thing sets me off.
- I feel as taut as an over-tuned violin string.
- I seem to have lost the ability to feel or to care for anything or anyone.

If you have ticked any in *My mind* or in *My emotional life* or have ticked more than one in *My social life* or two in *My body* then read on, because you are indeed stressed. At the start of this chapter we said that stress is all about living healthily and happily and staying alive. And indeed it is.

We can beat heart disease
Stress is a potent factor in coronary heart disease (CHD) which is the major killer of the industrialised West. The United Kingdom (Scotland, Northern Ireland, England and Wales) has had a seventeen per cent increase since 1980, most of this (twelve per cent) being in Northern

Ireland, naturally enough. The lowest figures in the West are for Switzerland. This may be because the opposite conditions to those in Northern Ireland apply. It has no warring or religious factions. It is a much more stable community and, being neutral, has fewer problems with its NATO and European neighbours. Can we in Britain bring these figures down? Yes we can if we begin to change our lifestyle. Until ten years ago the United States had the highest death rate from coronary heart disease in the world. They have reduced it by over thirty per cent. Look at this report from *Time* magazine, dated 31st March 1961, about the state of anxiety then rampant in the States:

'Anxiety threatens to become the dominant cliché of modern life. It shouts from the headlines, laughs nervously at cocktail parties, nags from advertisements, speaks suavely from the board room, whines from the stage, clatters from the Wall Street ticker, jokes with fake youthfulness on the golf course. Not merely the black statistics of murder, suicide, alcoholism, and divorce betray anxiety (or that special form of anxiety which is guilt), but almost any innocent, everyday act: the limp or overhearty handshake, the second packet of cigarettes or the third martini, the forgotten appointment, the stammer in mid sentence, the wasted hour before the TV set, the spanked child, the new car unpaid for.'

It is all too familiar to us today, isn't it? But our American cousins started doing something about it. They began to tackle stress in their workplaces, in their homes and in their personal lives. They began to change their lifestyle. They began to change their eating habits and whole grain cereals became popular while less junk food and more vegetables were eaten. They began to exercise in earnest and there are now eighteen million joggers in the States. And those who are not jogging are swimming, cycling or playing tennis. And what they have achieved I am perfectly certain we can achieve on this side of the Atlantic. But a word of warning to all you unfit people: do not go out jogging tomorrow. Read Chapter 11 first.

Living is a great deal more than just staying alive. Just staying alive can mean existing as an emotionally dried up automaton – drifting through life, but uninvolved in it. Life

Living is more than staying alive

17

is like this for a large number of people. Once one starts researching the extent of anxiety, depression, fears and phobias in our society today, the apparent size of the problem is alarming. To give you some idea: we top the poll of neurotics running a higher risk of mental illness (our rate is 355 per thousand population) than any of our more ebullient and volatile European neighbours. I can hear you asking, 'What exactly is a neurotic? I'm sure I'm one, or even a psychotic. I'm always afraid about something.' You are probably neither. Normal people from time to time have fears and worries, and are often anxious, resentful, suspicious or jealous. There lies the difference. The neurotic is in that state most of the time, and it colours his whole life. This makes him a desperately unhappy person.

Normal, neurotic or psychotic?

The psychotic on the other hand, is not in touch with reality at all. One small illustration may indicate the difference between the normal, the neurotic and the psychotic. Taking on a new job with new and different responsibilities makes many of us nervous and apprehensive. We may have a sleepless night or two, indigestion, and many visits to the loo: in fact, all the signs of stress. That is absolutely normal. The neurotic at this stage, however, is sure that he is ill and cannot possibly go and rings up to say that he is too ill to get out of bed. There he stays for a few days worrying about his health and he never does take up the job. The psychotic, on the other hand, withdraws from reality completely, and retreats into a world of his own. He is never going to get up or talk to anyone because he does not believe that life is worth living. Here is another illustration of the difference between the neurotic and the psychotic. There is a newspaper report that the sun is shrinking.
Normal reaction: 'Well, it will probably last my lifetime.'
Neurotic reaction: 'The world will get colder, there will be another ice age, what will happen to us all?'
Psychotic reaction: 'I know. I've been blowing it out.' The vicious circle of neurosis is that neurotic parents tend to make neurotic children. On the other hand, a warm, loving, outgoing relative, friend or teacher, can break this pattern. The drive which we all possess towards healthy growth, given half a chance, will help the child to develop normally. Our drive towards normality is very strong.

Anxiety and depression

Well over half the visits of patients to their family doctors are for help for the 'minor affective disorders' (anxiety and

18

depression to you and me). These two conditions are the result of stress. Anxiety is one of the commonest symptoms, and about one in ten adults see their doctor during the course of a year for anxiety, tension, or anxiety-related physical symptoms. (See chapter 14, *Understanding and coping with anxiety*.) Depression affects more women than men and about one in five see their doctor each year for this complaint. Eight million prescriptions are written annually for anti-depressants alone. (See Chapter 13, *Understanding and coping with depression*.) The most serious consequence of depression is suicide. In greater London alone there are about three every day. It is more common among men, but the rates for women are rising. It is thought that over five thousand people commit suicide in the UK every year which is more than half the number who die in road accidents.

These figures are bad enough, but they are only the tip of the iceberg, because many of us, ashamed at not being able to cope with our emotions, swallow a couple of aspirins, have another coffee or a strong drink, hoping that it will all just go away. The number of people suffering from mild obsessions (checking every hour or so that you really have turned the gas off) and phobias seem to be on the increase to judge from the letters which pour daily into the office of every problem page editor. Many of these letters contain an apology for being 'stupid', 'unable to cope with life' or not being able to 'snap out of it'. Anxiety just is not something one can 'snap out of' nor is depression something that will disappear when your family say, 'For heaven's sake smile, you are walking around like a wet week.' You look miserable because you are miserable, and if you are feeling down you cannot suddenly feel happy and smile to order. Not until your worries and problems have been sorted out. And what you need, to do that, is help, not brick-bats which make you feel worse.

Feeling down

As for an inability to cope, you have probably been coping only too well and trying too hard for too long a time. This striving against all odds keeps the pressure high and gradually exhausts you. It drains the body of all its reserves of energy. Building up these reserves again will take a little time but you can start the upward journey today and within a few weeks you will be smiling again and you will be able to toss those pills into the bin sooner than you think.

Coping too well

19

What is health? But living a full life once more does not mean living without stress. A little stress, as we shall see, gives us that get-up-and-go feeling. It provides the excitement, the 'high' of meeting a challenge and the exhilaration of riding the crest of the wave. Our problems and difficulties will still occur. The difference will be that we will be fit enough to take them in our stride once more, and have the resilience to make the decisions and to take action and deal with them. So how do we get fit and regain the energy and resilience to conquer all again? One hears a great deal about relaxation and meditation, but the most important way seems to be a well-kept secret. That secret is balance. We have to keep a balance in our mental health, in our social health and in our physical health. But most important of all, we have to keep a balance between all three. A tall order? Yes, it is, but it is amazing how simply it can be done when you begin to think about it and to apply some basic rules.

You see, good health is all about wholeness. The very word health itself means wholeness. It comes from our own old Anglo-Saxon word *hal, hael* or *hul* (they were not too pedantic about spelling in those days) meaning whole, together with the suffix *th* meaning in a state of. So we get *health* which means in a state of wholeness. Think about it – a whole and well balanced individual. That is health. Well balanced individuals make for a healthy, safe society.

A healthy balanced society? No, we are not balanced. We are a most unbalanced society. Principally because as individuals we are not balanced emotionally. We have a population largely drugged by tranquillisers and anti-depressants by day, and by sleeping pills at night. We have heroin addicts, alcohol addicts, work addicts and those addicted to sweets. Our consumption of sweets (challenged only by the USA) is the highest in the world. We buy them when we feel deprived or 'down'. We could say that we are becoming emotionally sterile. Whatever happened to happiness and plain common or garden contentment? Everyone you speak to is bored unless actively going somewhere to be entertained, and that costs money. Real pleasure, the pleasure of contentment, does not cost a thing. I remember watching a three-year-old in the train squealing with delight at the sight of lambs in a field. I looked, really looked, at them for the first time for years, and shared her delight.

20

But there is worse than boredom abroad in our midst. *A dangerous*
There is a dangerous malcontent on our streets and in our *discontent*
cities, which leads to aggression and violence. It is not
confined to England and is very much worse in other areas
of the industrialised West. What is it about industrial
societies that makes for violence? England was at its most
violent during the upheavals just before, during, and in the
years immediately following the industrial revolution. A
great deal of it is due to stress. We have not yet fully
appreciated the depths of despair, or the high aggravation
and frustration, that can build up to a level where an
explosion of aggression is a relief. Once indulged in, this
relief is sought again and again.

Sometimes aggression is seen in the them-and-us con-
frontation over a strike or a lock-out. It finds an outlet in
the differences between social groups in a community, or in
the relations between police and demonstrators. It can
result in a general feeling of irritability and intolerance
which finds an outlet in the home in wife-beating and child
abuse. Violence has its seeds in festering discontent. To
negate it in the next generation we must now set out
actively to foster contentment. And contentment is not
found by just improving the material environment. This
has been tried. We have developed the Welfare State – a
free Health Service, a minimum wage for all whether
employed or not, pensions, housing and high standards of
hygiene for all. Where then does contentment lie?

In most industrialised societies we have developed effort *Always striving*
and striving into a way of life. There is no longer a
contentment with what we are and what we have got. Our
children must be seen to be cutting their teeth early,
walking before others of their age and talking from the
cradle – or we think they are letting us down. We are not
content with what they are in themselves. They may be
budding artists or musicians or marvellous craftsmen who
excel with their hands. No, we insist that they do well
academically and then we wonder why they develop one or
other of the stress ailments – a stutter, eczema, hay fever or
asthma. Some become rebels or drop-outs, resentful and
discontented. Why do we not value and enjoy what they
are and what they have to give? We could help them
to develop to their fullest potential and to live contented, happy lives. We would certainly keep them alive
longer.

21

Stress in a consumer society

A part of the striving to have is fostered by the approach of advertising – which means that they find our weak spots. Try this game. Cut out pictures in advertisements without the name of the product. Mix them up and then try to find out what they are persuading you to buy. Not the ravishing blonde. Not the drop-head Ferrari. Probably just Brand X cigarettes. We buy the image. I am now resisting all blandishments, being content with what I have got and determined not to be seduced into buying gadgets which cost the earth, which are not designed to last, and which certainly do not reduce my stress. The old dolly and the wash tub of our grandmother's day was a great way to reduce stress. Even better is the old carpet beater. If you can find one, try it on a rug thrown over a washing line in the garden. It is magic for lessening tension and restoring one's temper and equilibrium. Pressing an electric button just does not have the same effect.

Getting the balance right

We have to begin to get our whole balance together again and then to live life as a whole person, not just functioning on one cylinder or in only one gear. Of course we are going to be thrown and knocked about by an engine that is neither balanced nor running smoothly, but we can get the balance right. The term mental health covers both our emotional health and our intellectual health. The seat of both is in the brain, and both are essential for a well balanced person. For example, if we are emotionally insecure, highly anxious or deeply depressed, we cannot develop our intellectual capabilities to the full. One affects the other. Our social health is vital to us in giving us the ability to develop friendships, and deeply satisfying personal relationships. Today these have to take the place of the family of old. That was a very large circle of blood relatives, relations by marriage, and all their friends. Our balance of physical health is vital to the healthy functioning of both mental and social health. It is, as it were, the solid foundation stone.

Fit or fit to drop?

Many of us believe that if we are able to walk, run to catch a bus without collapsing, and still do a day's work, we are fit. We may actually be very unfit. Real physical fitness can be seen and felt in, for example, the tingling glow we feel after a swim. It is different from the driven feeling of high arousal caused by stress, even though both can make one feel 'high' and exhilarated. The first is like the glow of

22

happiness, the second a burning fever. The first is the foundation for the balance of intellectual, emotional and social health. Our system is fully interdependent. In addition, we need to develop the health of the spirit, our quiet contemplative renewing of our inner selves. For this we need to develop time and space in which to be ourselves, wholly apart from the daily pressures. A surprisingly short time each day will do it. Think of yourself now as you can and will be – a whole, balanced, functioning, interactive, vital you.

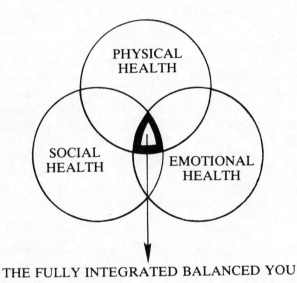

THE FULLY INTEGRATED BALANCED YOU

CHAPTER 2

Getting to grips with stress: What is it?

What exactly is stress?

If we have a thorough understanding of something, we are more likely to be able to deal with it. One of the disappointments in much of the writing on stress is that the issue of exactly what it is, has been ducked. This is understandable because it is a complex subject, and many writers would say, 'People don't want to know what it is, they want to be told how to cope with it.' One of the difficulties is that stress has never really been defined satisfactorily. The founding father of the subject, Professor Hans Selye (pronounced *shell-yea*), who died recently, was a Czechoslovakian. When writing his research papers for publication he relied upon an English friend for the word he wanted, and was given 'stress'. With his later command of the language he knew that the word stress was wrong – he should have used 'strain'.

Should it be 'strain'?

That makes very much more sense. Further difficulties were that his research on animals stressed them physically and they reacted by an overall generalised physiological response similar to that of 'fight or flight'. So, ever since those early days in 1936, when his research began to be published, we have been bedevilled by the word 'stress' and the idea of that generalised response. We now know that it is a very variable response and that physical and emotional stessors produce quite different reactions. We also know that different emotional states have their different chemicals, for example, those for anger and those for high irritation.

However, these difficulties do not entirely explain the very different interpretations put upon stress or strain by the media. They range from 'Stress is good for you' to 'Stress – the hidden killer'. Small wonder that we are confused.

24

Every book and every article meant for the general public perpetuates the myth that stress is simply the fight or flight reaction of the human body, and that we must control it and use it for our own energy needs. Can you imagine a complex interactional system like ours, capable of self-repair and of adaptation from the speed of the mule to that of the space shuttle in one generation, preserving intact without updating, a system developed for eluding dynosaurs, unless it was absolutely necessary to maintain it as it was? No, the picture of stress is very much more complex than this. We do have the 'fight or flight' reaction (the fully Automatic Primary Stress Response), but we also have Secondary Stress Responses which are not fully automatic but are set off by our thinking brain and by our emotional needs. Let us take the Automatic Primary Stress Response first.

Not just 'fight or flight'

This is a very fast defence reaction, often called the fight or flight response, caused by a reflex sympathetic nervous system discharge. Like other reflex actions in the body, it occurs faster than thought and it is the primary response to physical threat. The sympathetic nervous system is a part of the autonomic nervous system (that part which is not under conscious control). This system keeps our internal balance on an even keel, and is closely concerned with our biological clocks. Extreme demands from the environment, like a maniac about to attack us, or a lorry jack-knifing in front of us on the motorway, in fact any physical threat where our safety depends upon instantaneous reaction, is met by this system much quicker than we could plan a response ourselves.

The Automatic Primary Stress Response

An example of this physiological response in action once happened with me on a motorway. An articulated lorry jack-knifed in front of me. Before I could thoroughly appreciate the situation with my mind, I found myself pulled up on the shoulder within inches of three other cars and out of the way of the lorry which now straddled the three lanes ahead. A few seconds before we had been travelling at some seventy miles an hour in our separate lanes. One's reaction was almost instantaneous and there was certainly no time to have thought out what to do.

Another example of when this fight or flight mechanism switches on is when we have to undergo a major operation. It switches on to help the body over the shock of the surgery. So it will be obvious that this Automatic Primary

Stress Response is a life saver and is wholly good, and one would not want to control it or manage it in any way. It works perfectly, as most of our physiological reflexes do, even though in modern times it may not be in daily use. So stress is partly this automatic primary response. But if only partly, what is the rest? The rest is what we could call the Secondary Stress Response.

The Secondary Stress Response

This is a very complex pattern of both nerve and chemical reactions which the brain initiates from what it senses we need. While the fight or flight response is initiated probably from the arousal system in the brain stem, it is pretty certain that the variable Secondary Stress Response originates in different brain areas – the cognitive (thinking) brain when increased energy is needed for the things we want to do and accomplish, and the emotional brain centres (Limbic system) when differing emotions such as anger, distress and anxiety, raise the stress response.

Thinking and feeling is involved

As mentioned earlier, different patterns of biochemicals are mobilised in answer to different needs. For example, in anger or high irritation, the brain will mobilise much more Nor Adrenalin than Adrenalin, which is a fighting pattern. Further, it is not just an all-or-nothing response. Amounts varying from very small to very large can be mobilised, giving us from zero levels of energy up to very high peaks. Zero levels and below will be experienced in depressive states, and very high peaks in conditions known as Hypo Mania where body and brain are so highly activated that sleep and rest are impossible. It is these differing patterns of biochemicals which respond to our emotional state that we have to try to understand and control. These are best exemplified by the following expressions which we use every day:

> 'I want to,' 'I have to,' (I am being pressured to) and 'I can't escape from.'

Let us take the first of these.

'I want to'

If we are rehearsing for a play, maybe professionally or in an amateur capacity or at school, and we want desperately to do it, and do it well, we will be given the energy, strength and alertness to stay up all night if necessary to learn the part. How? We have an alert and vigilant system in the brain stem (the Ascending Reticular Arousal System or

26

ARAS for short) that can keep us awake until whatever it is that we desperately want to do is achieved. The consequent satisfaction is highly pleasurable and motivating. So the stressors involved in carrying out what 'I want to' do are well coped with. It is a wholly good form of stress if we do not keep up the pressure to the exclusion of our physical health.

This may be due to pressures imposed upon us by our work, by society, or by our family; for example in having too many responsibilities at work, having difficult situations at home with illness or rebellious teenagers. The chemicals mobilised depend upon how anxious or depressed we get in these situations.

'I have to' (I am being pressured to)

This state is the worst pattern of all. If we feel trapped, or feel that no matter what we do there is no escape from very stressful circumstances – for example, living with a drunken, bullying husband, or having the responsibility of a very seriously handicapped child, or living with the constant danger of mugging – the brain, feeling the needs from its emotional centres, will mobilise steroids (the big guns of the chemicals) to help us over these difficulties. They are meant to be helpful but have damaging effects on our health if kept up for too long because they interfere with our immunity and other defence systems. But if the brain believes that we are in a desperate fix it would rather settle for a gastric ulcer than extinction.

'I can't escape from'

These secondary stress responses are the ones we do need to control and manage. We need to be able to know and understand them and recognise them in ourselves, in our colleagues, staff, friends and relations. Some of these states are very good and useful to us, giving us extra power and energy when we most need them, providing we are able to control them when we do not actually need them.
   Others are potentially damaging to health. I can almost hear you say that the whole thing sounds very complex. Well, yes, it is, and there is a great deal that we do not yet know about the many hundreds of chemicals involved. So how can we understand it? We can understand it by first showing how the Automatic Primary Response mobilises the power and energy to enable us to do things like leaping twelve feet into a tree to escape a charging rhino when we couldn't normally jump a five-barred gate.

How can we understand this complexity?

27

How the Automatic Primary Stress Response works	When we see a threat to life, like that charging rhino, or hear drumming hooves behind us, it is thought that the Ascending Reticular System, our Vigilance for Danger system in the brain stem, trips the switch of the tiny packet of chemicals in a part of the brain called the mesenchephalon, which produces the Automatic Primary Stress Response. This is the integrating centre for both nerve and chemical information on the need for rapid mobilisation of energy for help in situations of emergency, threat, acute need, and, in fact, any situation which is likely to throw our system out of balance. In order to produce the Automatic Primary Stress Response, a massive discharge occurs from our Activating Nervous System (the Sympathetic Nervous System) which speeds us up.
Power, speed, energy	This activating system and the chemical system, acting together, provides us with the power, energy and speed to escape from most life-threatening situations where survival depends upon speed. The full pattern of what happens in the body and brain, showing the changes brought about by the Automatic Primary Stress Response which gives us extra power, speed and energy, is:-

Heart	The heart rate is speeded up giving a faster heart beat.
Blood pressure	This is raised to increase the circulation.
Blood vessels	There is a mechanism which makes blood clot so that when we are injured we do not lose it all. This clotting facility is increased in stress.
Circulation	This is increased to the brain for faster co-ordination. It is also increased to the muscles, particularly in the limbs, to power them for action.
Lungs	These are stimulated to make breathing faster and to quicken the oxygenation of the blood.

28

Liver	This releases sugar stores for quick energy.
Stomach	Digestion is stopped and the blood normally needed for this purpose is diverted to the limbs to power them for action.
Kidneys intestines and bladder	Their function is stopped, so fluid drainage from the kidneys is interfered with, the muscles at the openings of the bladder and anus are relaxed, often with embarrassing consequences.

All of these changes give us extra power and energy to deal with a threat to our equilibrium, and are, of course, only very temporary. When the emergency is over, we experience pounding heart, shaking limbs and sickness, as the body rights itself and the circulation returns to the stomach and intestines. The system returns to normal quickly and we are none the worse, except for a sick feeling at the thought of what might have been. As we said earlier, this response is a magnificent life saver. It is physiologically perfect, and we certainly do not need to alter it in any way. What we are much more concerned with is the secondary stress response and this is by far the more complex state to understand. We can understand it best if we break the whole process down into three stages – Stage I Stress: The mobilisation of energy, Stage II Stress: The consuming of energy and Stage III Stress: The draining of energy.

Stage I Stress – Mobilising energy

We have already seen in the Automatic Primary Stress Response how energy is mobilised in the system, but in considering the Secondary Stress Response we need to point out that there are different physical responses. In Stage I the stress triggers or stressors are different. In the 'I want to' situation, which is initiated by the thinking part of the brain (the cognitive system), the amount of energy mobilised is coped with mainly by the activating system together with the biochemicals Adrenalin, Nor Adrenalin

'I want to'

29

and Dopamine, with possibly Met Encephalon and Beta Endorphin. The exact proportions and mixtures of these chemicals are still unknown.

High motivation   In other words, there is a desire or high motivation to achieve and succeed for which there is a need for energy over and above the normal level needed for quiet everyday activity. The drive that gives rise to this can be an underlying need for status, a need to be recognised as a power or authority, a need to do a good job for one's own satisfaction, or the need to be seen to be better or more efficient than others. That felt high drive or need is a stress trigger causing that packet of chemicals (the overall stress response) to tip over and alert the activating system which in turn stimulates the production of Adrenalin and the release of the other chemicals mentioned above.

Emotional stress   The stress triggers can also be social stressors like a row
is high   with a neighbour or the boss. They can also be emotional stressors like the threat of a breakdown in a love affair.

We are astonishingly sensitive to emotional stress. The threat of something about to happen which can affect us emotionally is far more of a stressor than the actual happening. So the threat of a partner walking out of a marriage or a love affair, the threat of punishment to a child and the threat of redundancy, all can cause greater emotional distress than when it actually occurs. In distress, different chemicals are involved in the following way. When we make a conscious effort as in 'I want to', like someone studying for A levels or someone running his own business, we mobilise Adrenalin together with other stress chemicals. When we make a conscious effort to cope with a distressing situation like that of an over-worked and over-burdened housewife, we mobilise the bigger guns of Cortisol from a different part of the Adrenal gland, the Cortex. How can you recognise the Secondary Stress Response in Stage I Stress in yourself?

Signs of Stage I   Very easily, through the speeding up of all activity.
You act rather as if you had an over-active thyroid.
   You walk faster than usual.
   You talk and laugh more readily.
   You think much more rapidly, reach decisions and act much faster.
   You eat faster – often taking a sandwich on the job.

30

CHALLENGE	THREAT
MAKING EFFORT WITH SATISFACTION	MAKING EFFORT AND DISTRESSED
BRAIN'S COGNITIVE SYSTEM (Thinking)	BRAIN'S LIMBIC SYSTEM (Emotional)
STRESS RESPONSE	STRESS RESPONSE
	PITUITARY GLAND
SYMPATHETIC NERVOUS SYSTEM	A.C.T.H. (Adrenocorticotrophic Hormone)
ADRENAL MEDULLA	ADRENAL CORTEX
ADRENALIN	CORTISOL
SPEED AND ENERGY INCREASE	DISTRESS
EFFORT + SATISFACTION	*EFFORT + DISTRESS*

This is a diagramatic view of the difference between expending effort creating satisfaction, and expending effort creating distress. It is the difference between a challenge we enjoy and a threat to the system.

You drink faster – and leave many half-empty cups of tea or coffee as you have not taken the time to drink a whole one – and savour it.
You feel under pressure of time.
You feel as if you are being driven (which you certainly are – by the activating system).
But it is important to note that in the 'I want to' situation you feel great. You are achieving things faster. You are full of energy (literally) and feel that you have the power to

conquer the world; and of course you have. But remember that the extra energy you are demanding, if excessive, comes from other parts of the system. For example, take digestion. If you feel very motivated to succeed, you will not want to take the time to eat, and will not feel hungry. Yet you will need to eat in order to keep up the pattern of energy you are demanding. For this reason, working breakfasts or lunches should be kept to a minimum if you are highly involved in the working part of them.

You can recognise Stage I stress in others by their speeded up system which causes a faster pattern of activity, especially in walking and talking, and also by their excitable manner.

Stage I Stress: Good or bad?

Wholly good, because it is only a short-term stage and very useful if:

> You need to take rapid decisions or action in an emergency.
> You need all-out action in sports (for which you have trained in order to avoid damaging muscles or heart)
> You are going to an all-night disco (you should train for this too – you might slip a disc!).
> You have to meet an altered deadline which needs speed, all-out effort and the ability to keep awake for twenty-four hours.
> And in so many other circumstances when you need quick energy and an alert mind.

It is not an all-or-nothing response

At this point it is essential to reiterate one statement. It is not an all-or-nothing response like the Automatic Primary Stress Response. I know many books give this impression, but it is not true. The actual stress response (ie the amount of chemicals shot into the system) depends upon a number of factors. It depends firstly on how we ourselves think of the stressor – whether we see it as only vaguely annoying, or as disastrous. It depends also on how and when it occurs. A single stressor like a broken leg can be taken in one's stride at the age of eighteen with very little response, but at eighty-one a similar misfortune means nervous system involvement in a long-term and difficult problem, and generates much more response. On the other hand, the broken love affair at the age of seventeen is the end of the world and the response could be enormous and cause high

32

arousal levels. At twenty-eight, with greater maturity, it is just the end of an affair, and maybe the start of something better, so the response might be slight. It also depends upon the resources available to the individual. Strong emotional and social support can reduce the arousal levels and allow the system to return quickly to normal.

A transient stage

Stage I Stress is a transient stage which is finished as soon as that deadline or row is over, when everything goes back to normal. That is why it is good, useful, and indeed essential, to life. However, if there is continuing stressor or ongoing series of crises, the stress response is kept on continuously, the changes do not revert to normal and you move into Stage II Stress.

STAGE I STRESS

THE MOBILISATION OF ENERGY

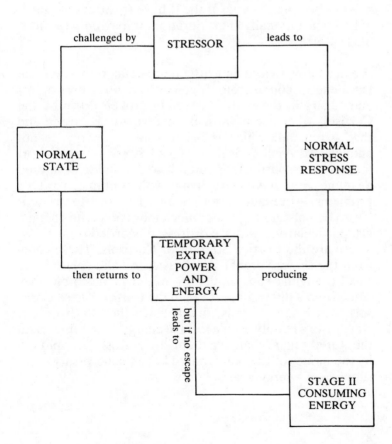

Stage II Stress – Consuming energy stores

'I have to' (I am being pressured to)

This is the stage of 'I have to' and 'I can't escape from'. The stress response is still on because you experience a continuous series of stress triggers. These may be, for example, working with a difficult boss who continually upsets you, having a problem at home with a rebellious son or daughter, or having the nuisance of noisy neighbours when you desperately need peace and quiet. Or it may just be the accumulation of small prickles both at home and at work. You have visitors arriving for the weekend, you have promised to have that long report ready on Monday morning, and the cat has 'flu. This you feel is typical of your life. Whatever the difficulties, if you feel distressed, the stress response will pick up the signals coming this time from your emotional centres in the brain and will immediately switch on and stay switched on in an effort to keep you well supplied with the extra energy and power it thinks you need to be able to cope. If the 'I have to' Stress trigger is only of exceptionally short duration, it may only result in Stage I Stress

When adrenalin is not enough

We need now to look in a little more detail into where the extra energy comes from. It comes from our stores of fats and sugars in the body. These are broken down by the Cortisols when the brain feels that we are distressed and that Adrenalin, which is just a shot of energy, is not enough. Adrenalin, ideal for Stage I Stress, is only a short term booster, particularly suitable to that suddenly altered deadline. But if you are living with continual rows or problems, Adrenalin is not enough. For long term use it has to be bolstered by other much more powerful chemicals, particularly if you are distressed, worried or anxious. These are the Cortico Steroids or Cortisols. These come from the same Adrenal glands as Adrenalin (placed like small triangular caps on the top of our kidneys) but they come from a different part called the Cortex. These Cortisols, which are steroids, break down the fats from our stores into a readily usable form of energy. They also act on the stored sugars changing them into glucose for rapid use by the tissues of the body. All to keep the necessary extra supplies of energy available.

34

What happens to all those rapidly mobilised fats and sugars? We are now far less physical than we were even a generation ago. Most children then walked miles to school and adults often walked five or six miles a day or more. Today, most workers are sedentary, or at best standing tending the machines that do the hard physical labour. So we no longer have the same need for all this extra power and energy. We may be just sitting fuming in a traffic jam, or sitting at a desk striving to make the next deadline. If the stress triggers keep the Secondary Stress Response on, the extra fats and sugars are not converted back into stores. This only happens when the system is allowed to return to normal. They have been changed into fatty oils and glycerols and together with numerous other chemicals and hormones they circulate in the bloodstream.

Where does the power and energy go?

STAGE II STRESS

CONSUMING ENERGY

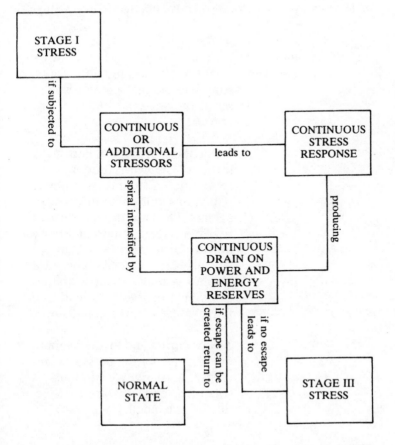

The fats stay in the bloodstream

If they are neither used up nor stored, the danger is that the fats will attach themselves to the walls of our arteries damaging them. The chemicals and the residue, if the oils remain uncombusted, will silt up the body cells and inhibit their normal healthy function. So they are indeed dangerous to our health, but they can be got rid of by the simple process of physical exercise. (See Part II, Chapter 11.) In Stage II Stress, to keep healthy, fit and energetic, you must burn up these extra fats and sugars to release from the cells the burden of unused chemicals which are making you feel fatigued and leading to feelings of anxiety. To feel really fit and well you must actively remove them from the body and brain. The best form is uncompetitive swimming which uses every muscle in the body, or brisk walking in the open air at least once a day. Anxiety and tiredness will disappear and you will feel marvellous. Your cells will be able to work properly again, and you will soon sparkle with health and energy.

How can you tell when you have been too long in Stage II Stress?

Indulging in comfort tricks

1 Food: spicy food is sought or something exotic and different to stimulate fading palates. Sweets, particularly chocolate, are craved.

2 Alcohol: drink is taken for a lift and, as with food above, something different is sought. (Cocktails will come into vogue again!) The one drink to try to revive a flagging mind and body quickly turns into two or three. As problems recede (because alcohol is really an anaesthetic) drinking to forget can lead one fairly quickly into alcoholism.

3 Sex: caring and loving begin to fall off as stress pressures increase, so extra stimulus is sought. (Sex shops are a reflection of this need.)

4 Tobacco: smoking increases, the amount often doubling during stress.

Feeling driven   You will feel driven and indeed you are being driven by the activating system which is still switched on.

Time pressures   As you begin to lose energy towards the end of this stage you will feel over aware of time pressures and of a high workload.

Tiredness and fatigue   You take a long time to go to sleep and wake earlier than usual.

Memory   Towards the end of this stage, memory begins to let you down.

Anxiety   This develops as you begin to notice your lack of drive and energy. You cannot continue at the same over-high pace you have been setting yourself.

Ill-health   Twitching legs and cramps: these become frequent at night.
Stomach difficulties: gastritis, dyspepsia and stomach cramps can develop through over-rich and spicy food when normal digestion is stopped by stress.
Tension headache and Migraine: a tension headache is often felt as a tight band around the skull. Migraine may also develop.

How do you recognise it in others?

Smokers will very often double their usual intake. Drinkers will consume more alcohol and there will be evidence of this in the office and in the lunchtime sessions, and after work in the evening. There will be a tense set to the shoulders and head, and irritation will become more evident.

37

*Personality
give-aways*

When the period has been going on for some time you will notice that their particular personality quirks and traits will be increased. For example, a person who is naturally tidy will become excessively so. If a pen has been moved two inches there will be an outburst. A person who is naturally greedy will become more so and overeat. A person who naturally has little interest in food will become more so and lose weight. A person who finds fault easily will become an absolute trial to work for. An individual who is normally quick tempered will seem to be always in a state of temper for no reason. The danger signals are the high irritation and quick flare-ups for very minor things, the over-reaction to every minor problem and increased personality traits.

*Not really
harmful unless*

This is not really a harmful stage unless it is accompanied by some distress. If it is, harmful chemicals will be circulating in the system, and if at the same time you are consuming more energy from your stores than you are replacing during rest and sleep, then your whole system will become strained. You will then drift into Stage III Stress which is the harmful strained stage. It is therefore of the utmost importance that you recognise when this stage has been going on for too long. You will notice that the pattern of your life is changing. Your sleep patterns will become disturbed – not just on the occasional night, but as a regular pattern. You will find yourself constantly reacting with irritation at things to which you would previously have paid no attention. You will be uptight and taut, which will cause you to flare up in anger frequently.

The Real Danger Signals

The signals that Stage II Stress is going on too long are:

1 An alteration in your usual sleep patterns, (usually waking up at 4am or 5am after having taken two to three hours to get off to sleep).

2 Bouts of irritation becoming increasingly the principal way in which you react to problems.

3 Flare-up of anger at very minor things to which you would normally pay no attention.

4 Over-reaction to every minor difficulty.

5 Very occasionally, in some people, there is such a winding up and such a high level of arousal that it leads to mania – that is, everything is done at a highly excitable top speed. The body and mind are 'driven' and no sleep or rest is taken for days on end. High sedation then is absolutely essential to bring the system back to normal.

These are all signs (and your family and colleagues will know them) that Stage II Stress has gone on for too long and alterations have to be made if you are not to slip into Stage III Stress. Look very carefully at these signs and if you have even two out of the five danger signals listed above, stop now, take stock of your life before you drift into Stage III Stress, and illness.

In taking stock you have to look very carefully at the balance in your life. Health is not just the absence of disease or keeping on with the assertion that, 'I've never had a day off in my life.' It comes from a positive balance between emotional health, intellectual health, social health and physical health. In high stress arousal you will find that this balance is missing. Check for yourself how badly your balance is out, and what needs to be done to restore it to normal.

Taking Stock and Stopping Stage II Stress

Emotional Health How many times lately have you:			
	often	*not often*	*rarely*
1 Really laughed – full belly laughs of pure enjoyment?			
2 Shown really deep caring affection for your friends?			
3 Re-created your emotional depths of feeling with some personal experience of music, whichever type moves your spirit?			
4 Enjoyed satisfying sexual relationships with your partner?			

Social health

How many times lately have you:

	often	*not often*	*rarely*
1 Entertained your friends (other than business), even for only coffee and talk?			
2 Been in contact with friends who live far away?			
3 Been in contact with *all* your family?			
4 Contacted all your relatives?			

Family and relatives are still the major source of help when the going is a little tough, even though we may fight with them.

Intellectual health

How many times lately have you:

	often	*not often*	*rarely*
1 Felt really stimulated intellectually in your job?			
2 Enjoyed the stimulus of debating a subject with friends?			
3 Become involved in other interests outside your job?			

Physical health

How many times lately have you:

	often	*not often*	*rarely*
1 Sat down and enjoyed a good breakfast?			
2 Given time to relaxing the tension of the morning before you settle down to lunch?			
3 Walked up the stairs instead of taking the lift?			
4 Walked a brisk two miles?			
5 Been swimming, which exercises all the muscles of the body?			
6 Walked for five or ten minutes before bedtime?			

Look very carefully at the questions, see where your life is out of balance. You should be doing the majority of things often. If you are not, take out your diary now and plan in it the changes necessary to restore the balance.

Stage III Stress: Draining energy stores

Usually people have already reached this stage when they say 'I'm under stress' and go to their doctor for help. This is understandable because they are now feeling the effects of a body and brain which has been under strain for some time. That strain is beginning to tell, not only in their emotional health as shown by their increasingly high irritability and over-reaction to trifles, but also in their physical health as fatigue is felt. In their intellectual health concentration begins to fall off as the brain becomes drained of energy.

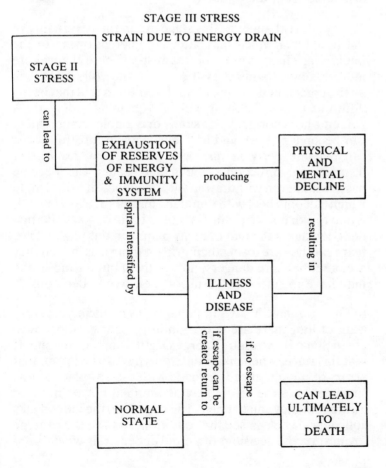

STAGE III STRESS

STRAIN DUE TO ENERGY DRAIN

Signs of energy drain

Just as with a car, whose owner has been too busy to have it serviced for a few years, the engine is sluggish. It does not react to the accelerator with the usual burst of speed. It is difficult to start in the morning and very slow to get going. It is clogged up with uncombusted fuel and has no oil. It is used up. So it is with our own system. Our accelerator is the stress response and we are not responding to it with our usual burst of speed – in fact, possibly no speed at all. We have a certain amount of resistance against 'getting going' and a feeling of deadness, rather as if one is clogged with cotton wool. One is clogged of course with all the residue of uncombusted biochemicals and in addition our energy stores are close to empty. Often the head feels larger than normal and stuffed with wadding and thinking through the wadding is difficult. Thoughts often circulate around problems which previously would have been solved quickly and dismissed from the mind.

Energy drain in the personality

The greatest changes at this stage are in the personality of the individual which may alter completely owing to the underlying changes in his biochemistry. These changes are more easily recognised by the family and colleagues than by the person undergoing them. Even when told that he is a different person lately it will be vehemently denied. A person who is normally of a sunny or equable temperament can become peevish and irritable. A once forceful leader can become petty in his ideas and lose all his former inspirational direction. A dynamic leader can become passive and even withdrawn. All is evidence of a tired mind which can only deal with mundane matters at a low level. It is due to exhaustive tiredness, not to brain damage. Permanent damage is the fear of many people in this plight. They fear that they are losing their grip on things, as indeed they are, and there are dangers, not for them but for those who may have to suffer the result of their wrong decisions.

Errors of judgement

In Government, in law, in industry, in medicine, in every walk of life, there are people in important positions who are in Stage III Stress or Energy Drain from time to time. It is at this stage, when major decisions have to be taken, that errors of judgment can be made with catastrophic results. In some cases the errors may be minimal but we must be aware that they can happen. The onus is on the individual's colleagues who can see the condition, to have the courage to question the decisions of a mind under strain which is too

42

tired to analyse all the known facts on which a correct decision can be made.

Signs of energy drain

*In physical
health*

Recurrent headaches.
Ringing in the ears or frequent head noises.
Frequent use of antacids or other self-prescribed drugs.
Palpitations and chest pain.
Frequent heartburn, stomach cramps, diarrhoea, being 'full of gas', unable to swallow.
Trembling under any extra pressure, leg cramps or pain, twitching in limbs.
Feeling that you may pass out.
Getting any illness that is around.

All are evidence of failing physical health.

*In intellectual
function*

Having a frequent thick cotton wool head (even without excessive alcohol).
Loss of former high concentration.
Loss of former reliable memory.
A new inability to reach satisfactory decisions.
New difficulty in thinking around problems.
New difficulty in dismissing problems from the mind.
Insomnia.

All are evidence of a tired mind.

*In emotional
health*

A feeling of being very low and dulled.
A shut-down in all emotions except anger and irritation.
All joy, laughter and pleasure have dried up.

43

Active love and caring have lessened or disappeared.
Tears seem frequently very near for no reason.

All are evidence of exhausted emotional health.

In others

The most important signs noticed are:

Change in personality: they become very difficult to live with.
Change in temperament: laughter, joking and fun disappear.
Quick anger for very trivial reasons.
Frequent complaint of headache.
Failing memory.
Difficulty in coming to a decision.
An obvious slowing down both mentally and physically.

It is as if the ageing process has suddenly overtaken them.

Is this 'Burn Out'?

Lately, in many magazines, there have been rather frightening references to something called 'Burn Out'. This is supposed to occur when the brain has become exhausted and 'is not able to function any more'. The person has 'burnt himself out', his intellectual functions have gone and he is left as a vegetable. Now, this is just nonsense, and highly stress-inducing nonsense at that. We have 10,000 million brain cells. We do not use one half of them, and even if we did there are cells in the brain which are regenerative (glial cells) and there are nerve endings quite capable of opening new pathways (synapses) in the brain. We can have a tired brain and even an exhausted brain which is unable to function because it needs rest in order to recuperate. We do not have 'burnt out' brains.

Charles – a case study

Our bodies (and this includes the brain) are very adept at telling us when they can cope no longer with the strains we are putting upon them. When they cannot cope any longer they stop. If it is the brain which has been overloaded

44

non-stop at the expense of the body, it is the body which will scream, as in the case of Charles, who worked at his desk almost night and day for four years. He took no breaks, no exercise, no relaxation – just work and little sleep. One day he found himself standing in front of his desk screaming. His doctor put him to bed and kept him there – thoroughly sedated for three days of absolute rest. Then he was gradually encouraged to develop a balanced routine, and he is now fully recovered. The human system is a very remarkable system indeed. It is self-regenerative and self-energising, but we have to keep a balance between its various functions if we are to remain healthy.

Unless stopped the body and brain will come to a standstill. The only way out is to take a break of at least two weeks and do absolutely nothing. Rest and sleep for the majority of this time. This is not a stage for exercise, but for rest and recuperation and for a clear re-assessment of the entire balance of your life. (See Chapter 9.)

The stages

Stage	Description	Resources mobilised	Symptoms
	The Self Generated Response		
STAGE I STRESS *Short-term mobilisation* (mobilising energy)	A. *'Fight or flight'* The unconscious and instantaneous response to imminent danger – chased by a bull, mugged.	Switching all energy from digestion, etc. to power limbs for action.	Fast speed, power and energy well above normal.
	B. *'I want to'* The conscious demand for extra energy for achievement – chasing a bus, meeting a deadline, achieving success.	Mobilising extra energy by increased heart beat, blood pressure, faster breathing, etc.	Energetic, exhilarated. Quickened action. Can stay awake and alert to finish a job.
	The Imposed Response		
STAGE II STRESS *Long-term mobilisation* (consuming energy)	C. *'I have to'* (I am being pressured to) The continuous consumption of energy reserves to meet imposed needs – commuting, heavy workload, difficult boss.	Fats, sugars and the stress chemicals mobilised for extra energy.	High energy and function. If prolonged this will decline.
	D. *'I can't escape from'* The excessive consumption of energy reserves to meet inescapable pressure – caring for a handicapped relative, living with a drunken spouse.	Steroids put out to keep system going. Conversion of stores of energy.	'Comfort tricks'. Irritability. Over-reaction to trifles.
	Distress and Illness		
STAGE III STRESS *Illness* (draining energy stores)	E. *'I am suffering from stress'* The exhaustion of energy stores with the consequent inability to meet pressures, leading to illness and possibly death.	Conversion of the ultimate reserves of energy.	Function slowing down. Memory and concentration go. Personality changes.

# of stress

Tiredness and function	Related illness	Exercise or rest	Assessment
Pant and feel sick. Trembling and slow afterwards.	None	Nil. Sit quietly and rest afterwards.	Wholly good reaction. Essential to life.
Pleasantly tired afterwards.	None as long as it really is short-term.	Normal aerobic exercise.	Good as long as it really is short-term.
Tiredness.			
Tiredness not relieved by sleep.	Anxiety Alcoholism Gastritis Depression	Aerobic activity essential with relaxation techniques to reduce arousal and tension.	Not harmful if accompanied by plenty of recreation, relaxation and rest, but potentially harmful.
Exhaustion.	Insomnia. Cardiac incidents. Hypertension. Personality problems. Physical or Mental breakdown.	Rest, sleep and holiday absolutely essential.	Wholly bad, leading to illness and ultimately to death.

CHAPTER 3

Why do we have so much stress in the 20th Century?

Society is less violent than in earlier centuries; plague, famine and poverty no longer destroy us, and we are more affluent, healthier and we live longer. Why then do we have so much stress today? There are many reasons for this. It is due partly to the society in which we live, partly to the way we live our lives within that society, and partly it is to do with us, and with the type of person we are. We are all individuals and react to stresses and strains in our own way. Some of these ways may even add to our stressors. So our stress triggers today are partly due to society, partly to the way we live, and partly to the way we are.

Stress due to society

Removal from our roots

To understand this we have to go back quite a long way to the changes initiated in the Industrial Revolution. The long-term effects of the changes that started then, and the speed of the technological revolution we are witnessing today, have together brought about the following changes in society:

1 Removal of people from their geographical roots in the countryside and small towns.
2 Removal of individuals from the economic security traditionally centered in the family.
3 Removal of individuals from their traditional social and emotional means of support.
4 The rapid growth in the population.

The small family unit

The distancing from our geographic, economic and social roots, has had far-reaching effects on both the family and the individual. It has resulted in the breaking down of the large and powerful family structure into small independent

48

mobile units of two adults and two children. Another result is that of loneliness. It is now rare for people to live in small settled societies, where everyone is known and where a stranger would be welcomed into the community. Our whole population is becoming mobile. People themselves move to find jobs or a better way of life in a different neighbourhood, or to retire at the end of a working life.

People are also moved by their employers – particularly by the large national and multi-national organisations. These have developed a policy akin to that of the armed services where people are moved on the average of every two years. This results in a varied life which may suit single people or childless couples, but it poses difficult problems for the shy. It also poses problems for families with children at secondary school. A mobile population tends to result in dormitory towns or suburbs with little community spirit or involvement. This makes for loneliness for the single young, the shy and the elderly. Families with very young children usually meet together through their children in nursery schools or play groups where there is more parent involvement. Lack of a community spirit is very hard on those who are not strong enough to forge their own relationships or develop friendships. One cannot just go up to a stranger and say, 'Will you be my friend?' There are so many strangers today.

A mobile population

Our population has grown from a fairly stable eight million before the Industrial Revolution to over fifty-five and a half million today. The stress triggers from this population growth stem from the fact that industrial cities have grown and extended their boundaries so quickly that in many cases they have coalesced to make what is called a conurbation. Forty per cent of the population of England and Wales now live in six large conurbations which total less than four per cent of the area of the British Isles. This makes for the stressors of traffic jams, rush hour, air pollution, the overstretching of all the health, housing and social services, and all the other problems associated with high population density.

Our over-crowding problem

Our present speed of technological change is without precedent. For example, before we had had time to get used to those colossal computers, let alone learn how to programme them, they were out of date. We now have

Skills are rapidly out of date

micro, and even mini, computers, which are available to all. The speed of change is such that if you are a secretary and leave your job for six months to have a baby, when you return you may find that the small word processor you had mastered with so many tears of frustration has been replaced by a micro computer. You will be expected to know how to work it after two easy lessons. And that may not be all. If you have a new junior she probably knows how to work it – she had one at school. These are the kinds of situations which are now only too familiar to us, and they are a potent source of stress.

Knowledge is now centered in the young

Our world is already different from that of our parents and grandparents, so there are ever widening gaps between our lifetime experiences and the world in which our children are growing up. This means that suddenly the knowledge and experience of one generation is neither useful nor acceptable to the next – yet another source of stress. Rapid changes in knowledge mean that people's omnipotence is quickly out of date. The younger and the more recently qualified a person is, the better he is at his job because his elders in that field cannot keep up with all the new techniques. Who would have thought a few years ago that someone's heart, lungs or liver could be taken out of one body, kept 'alive' and functioning properly, and then put in to work in someone else's? Or that small children would use computers in school. Or that there would be a shuttle service linking up with space stations. It all sounds like science fiction to those of us who are grown up, doesn't it? But not to our children. To them, these are the normal happenings of their world.

Our world has suddenly gone topsy turvy. Knowledge was always centered in the old. They had developed their skills and added the wisdom and experience of a lifetime's practice in them. They were venerated and the young would sit at their feet and listen and learn. Elders had status in the community, so also had doctors for their medical skills; teachers were respected for their knowledge; and the law was held in respect. Today all have lost their status. The skills of the old are unwanted, doctors are sued in the courts, learned judged are called to account, and teachers in state schools in inner city areas often have to cope with open rebellion. Parents used to have acknowledged authority in anything that concerned their children. Today we cannot even help them with their homework.

The result of the explosion of knowledge in many fields, and changing technology, is that nothing is any longer accepted as the one truth. Everything changes.

The speed and pace of change poses problems for the traditional transmission of acknowledged patterns of behaviour. In a settled and stable community the enduring values and beliefs which govern behaviour, are passed on from one generation to the next. Life is predictable. Everyone behaves in the expected way and there is security in the feeling and knowledge that this is how life is. Do we have any beliefs or values to pass on today? That seems questionable, like all our values. It is as if we are caught up in such a whirl of change that we question all previously held beliefs. Now most Western countries have populations of very mixed religions. They contain all the Western world's belief groups and many of the Eastern religions as well. Freedom of choice is a very good stress reducing principle. What is a cause of high stress, though, is the insecurity of the young who do not know what to believe in, if anything. Children, more than any other group in the community, need their world to be predictable and have to be able to rely on reality. Today, all the schools in the inner city areas have a large quota of disturbed children in every class. It is not surprising, but it is tragic nevertheless. But man is infinitely adaptable and we will survive, but we do need to understand what we are doing to the next generation in terms of their stress load. It is very, very high.

The speed and pace of external change

There has been a great deal of research into this question for some years now. The first systematic enquiry was made by Dr Adolph Mayer, a psychiatrist, in 1948. Then two American doctors, Holmes and Rahe, became interested in the question. They carried out extensive studies with many different groups of people all over the world. They set out the results of all their studies in a scale called the Social Readjustment Rating Scale. It has proved to be a reliable and valid indicator after more than twenty years of work with it and it holds true for many different cultures, both East and West.

How much change can we take?

Identify which of the following events have happened to you in the past year, and then add up the total Life Change Units scored.

The Holmes and Rahe Social Readjustment Rating Scale

Life events	Lifechange units
Death of spouse	100
Divorce	73
Marital separation	65
Imprisonment	63
Death of close family member	63
Personal injury or illness	53
Marriage	50
Dismissal from work	47
Marital reconciliation	45
Retirement	45
Change in health of family member	44
Pregnancy	40
Sex difficulties	39
Gain of new family member	39
Business readjustment	39
Change in financial state	38
Change in number of arguments with spouse	35
Major mortgage	32
Foreclosure of mortgage or loan	30
Change in responsibilities at work	29
Son or daughter leaving home	29
Trouble with in-laws	29
Outstanding personal achievement	28
Wife begins or stops work	26
Begin or end school	26
Change in living conditions	25
Revision of personal habits	24
Trouble with boss	23
Change in work hours or conditions	20
Change in residence	20
Change in schools	20
Change in recreation	19
Change in church activities	19
Change in social activities	18
Minor mortgage or loan	17
Change in sleeping habits	16
Change in number of family reunions	15
Change in eating habits	15
Vacation	13
Christmas	12
Minor violations of the law	11

This scale is useful as an indication of how much change you should allow in any one period of twelve consecutive months. Remember that the changes are cumulative during that period. When these life change units total 150–199 in any one year, this is a mild life crisis, and the medical histories of people in this bracket have shown that thirty-seven per cent had a subsequent appreciable deterioration in health. A total of 200–299 has proved to indicate a moderate life crisis, and in this group fifty-one per cent of research subjects examined had changes for the worse in their health. Over 300 indicates a major life crisis, and seventy-nine per cent in this bracket fell ill within the following year. *What is your score?*

If you are one of those like me, whose score is regularly bordering that 300 mark, remember that twenty per cent did not become ill. Your personality has to be taken into account (See Chapter 6). Consideration has also to be given to the way in which you personally handle change. If you have always revelled in change, and know when you have had enough you will be among the twenty per cent who will be alright. *How to interpret the results*

To understand how to cope with change and remain healthy, we must have some idea of how much change we are letting ourselves in for. For example, how much change in your life will marriage make? Or children? How much change is involved in moving house? Are these changes more or less stressful if you are a woman? How will buying a house for the first time affect you? It is worth working out in advance how stressful such changes are likely to be? For example, if your working life is currently undergoing a great deal of change, perhaps a change of management or structure, then leave any other changes until later and then carry them out one at a time. Let us look first at getting married – it makes for more changes than you would think, and it may well be different for men and women. *Change is cumulative*

Getting married if you are a man

Marriage	50
Change in financial state	38
Revision of personal habits	24
Change in sleeping habits	16
Change in eating habits	15
TOTAL	143

53

Getting married if you are a woman

Marriage	50
Change in financial state	38
Change to different work	36
Change in responsibilities	29
Change in living conditions	25
Revision of personal habits	24
Change in work conditions	20
Change in residence	20
Change in social activities	18
Change in sleeping habits	16
Change in eating habits	15
TOTAL	291

This pattern is different, of course, if you are already living and working together, when the act of marriage involves no change except a psychological one, and there certainly will be that.

Reduce stress in marriage

Every new adjustment to be made increases the load on the stress response and on our bodies and minds, so keep the changes as few as possible.

1 Look for your mates within your own circle of friends or in the place where you live or work.
2 Keep your two backgrounds as close as possible in how you have been raised.
3 Keep your two backgrounds as close as possible in your religion.
4 Keep your two backgrounds as close as possible in your value systems (what you believe to be important in a way of life).
5 Keep as similar as possible your ideas on having a family.

This is not to say that opposites do not find each other very stimulating, they usually do. Sometimes too much so for comfort! If you have a very demanding job with responsibilities for people – like a doctor, criminal lawyer, air traffic controller, policeman or probationary officer – you need stability and support to keep the stress triggers down, rather than someone who is a ball of fun at parties. On the other hand, if you have a routine, run-of-the-mill job at work, look for the stimulus in your life from your partner and your social life. Work out for yourself the cumulative scores for any changes you are about to make. If there is already a great deal of change in your life, think twice before adding to it. For example, if you are facing major upheavals at work or in your home life, keep all other changes to an absolute minimum. Do not even buy a cat. Learn to say No. It is a powerful way of reducing stress.

The family of old

This is the career we now need badly in our society. It is not for every woman, any more than child-bearing itself is. *Mother – the power in the home* Some will just not make good mothers. Anyone concerned with the breeding and rearing of animals will know this to be true. So why do we expect it to be so different in ourselves? Those who are life's natural good mothers can make an enormous contribution to the lowering of stress in our society if they could only be persuaded to take it on and put the family back in the place of priority over the workplace. Not so long ago the family was a very powerful institution and the mother the most powerful person in it. It has changed out of all recognition and, as well as leading to anxiety and insecurity in children, these changes account for many of our high stress triggers in parent/child and male/female relationships today.

Why was the family so powerful? It was powerful and had tremendous prestige through the functions that it had for all its members.

The family was its own banker, supplier, producer, marke- *Economic power* ter, and consumer. Marriage was of such vital economic and social importance that it could not be left to chance. Romantic love which comes and goes was thought to be a passing fancy and too risky a business altogether when considering the stability of the family and its future.

This featured in the home as apprenticeship for the skills *Education* needed to follow in the footsteps of the family. If secondary education could be afforded, a governess or a tutor was employed in the home.

The husband's physical prowess ensured the safety of his *Protection* wife and children. We had no police force until late in the last century.

55

TO35951

Caring for the sick	The mother attended to the care of the sick. She was both doctor and nurse. The knowledge of the treatment of ills, accidents and childbirth was handed down from mother to daughter and the women of the household. There were no fully trained nurses until the present century.
Religion	Religious belief was kept alive in the family by family prayers every morning, grace before every meal and readings from the Bible every evening after supper. Both parents usually had the same religious background. This continued until our grandparents' time. Today, the way-of-life religions have largely gone from the West except for Judaism and, to a lesser extent now, Roman Catholicism. Suicide and high stress are still lowest among members of these religious groups.
Status	All these functions (now taken over by the state) meant that membership of a family was of vital importance. It alone gave one status, work, economic security, friendship and protection. The family name was like a passport and one was known by it.
The affectionate bond	I have left this till last because as you can see, it is the only function now left to the family. It does not mean that the other skills are lost for they have been taken over by the State, but the state is not interested in us as individuals, and this is our greatest loss.
Partners or competitors?	**Men and women today.** It is said that the Equality Acts have given women the freedom of choice to train for and take up a career or to marry and have a family. The choices are not that clear cut, though, are they? Many girls go straight from school to college, fall in love and marry, have a baby, return to finish their studies and find themselves being girl friend, student, wife, lover and mother. It is small wonder that most married students taking their final examinations are also taking Valium. They are highly stressed. After their finals, they find themselves competing for jobs in the same market place as their husbands.
Single women and men	Also highly stressed are the single girls who want to settle down and have a family as well as a career – as the men are able to do – but who seem to meet only men intent on

56

affairs with 'no strings attached'. While it is cheaper today to share flats and each pay their own way, in between these affairs there are some very lonely, highly frustrated and highly stressed single girls.

Both sexes have their problems. Neither side really understands the other's needs physically or emotionally. Girls expect men to react like themselves and they do not. Men expect girls to react like men, and they do not. The sexes are very different in their attitudes to sex, love and marriage. The external positioning of their sexual organs creates in men a physical need for sexual release. They may have no emotional need at all, and this many girls simply do not understand. Girls more often associate sex with love and tend to become emotionally involved, feeling very confused when the man in their life at the moment seems to feel none of the same involvement. So the two sexes have quite a different approach to love which is largely un-voiced. So girls – start talking! You are so good at talking to each other, but it is the man in your life with whom you should be communicating; telling him how you feel and what your needs and desires are, and let him learn about women. Do not just silently wonder what his inmost intentions are.

The changes in society are making for rapid changes in the family and in marriage. Nearly half of all marriages now end in divorce, but there is now greater scope for men and women to become real partners in the rearing of their children, and this will no doubt continue to evolve. In the meantime, we are probably facing the highest degree of emotional stress resulting from the uncertainty and unpredictability of current male and female relationships. The old 'walking out – engaged – married' pattern was rigid and stultified, but it was a stable and predictable one.

Stress due to our culture

The protestant work ethic has served our country well. Because the puritans believed that work was good in the sight of God, the freemen of England did not lose face by working for a master for wages, and the Industrial Revolution gained its workers. However, the dictum reached unparalleled heights in Victorian England when, if you were not doing God's work, you were in danger of being got at by the Devil. There grew up the saying beloved by the Victorian mother 'Satan makes work for idle hands to

The protestant work ethic

do'. This has led to a society over-burdened with the guilt of those who are not busy all the time. Mothers tired out from fetching, carrying, ferrying, cooking and cleaning in the home, sitting having a breather for a moment, leap to their feet as if ashamed to be found doing nothing, the moment husband or children come home.

The guilt of inactivity

This constant activity is not of course bad in itself: it is the guilty feeling when one relaxes that is highly stressful, and takes away the very benefit of the relaxation. Husbands of working wives feeling that they should be helping with the household chores say, 'I'd just like to listen to the news, dear.' In reality, they want a ten-minute breather. One should be able to sit and wallow in the sheer delight of sitting doing absolutely nothing. Even our children are kept busy morning, noon and night.

Our achievement-orientated society

We have developed an achievement-orientated society with a 'busy' syndrome, but this drive can well lead to shortened lives. But, you will say, surely achievement is good? Everyone naturally wants to win and to do well? This is only too true, but not everyone can win or reach the top. There is far more stress in industrial societies just because they are based on the striving of the individual to master the skills needed to reach the top. Some societies (called closed) are based on what is called 'ascribed status' which means that who and what you are is determined at your birth together with your sex, race, colour, position, work and so on.

Not reaching the top

In open societies like ours, status depends upon the skills, knowledge, education, diligence and hard striving of the individual. Theoretically, everyone in an open or an industrialised society can become the President, the Prime Minister, professor of a university, chairman of a company or a millionaire. Conversely, this means that many of those who have set their sights on these goals must fail in the very fierce competition. Life for many inevitably becomes a long struggle with successive failures along the way. Some cannot face the damage that this does to their egos and they drop out of what has been called the rat race. All the stress triggers of frustration, anxiety and depression can affect us when we fail to reach our goals.

58

The British alone among the nations of the European Community seem to be ashamed of any outward show of emotion. I wonder what we British, in particular the middle classes, are doing to the next generation of lovers, husbands and friends? There is a myth embedded in the stiff upper lip tradition that real men do not like to be touched, let alone hugged and kissed, after the age of five. They do not like any show of emotion. All outward signs of love, affection and caring are withheld by the family, because 'boys don't like it'. How on earth are they supposed, spontaneously, to reverse this pattern some twenty years later and suddenly become tender, caring lovers, friends and husbands? No wonder many become overconcerned with their physical sexual prowess which, like their sports, can be kept at a purely physical level.

The stiff upper lip

Many countries have developed ways in which to handle their stresses. The poor countries have their feast days when the people dress in their best, parade, sing and dance, and for one glorious day are in a different world of gaiety and make-believe. The laughter and the dancing gives them great stress release, both emotionally and physically. And the date of the next one is already in the calendar to look forward to. The way that grief is handled by many other nations is a time-honoured ritual of mourning and weeping, often in the company of others. The wearing of special clothes proclaims your status, and you are allowed to grieve – indeed it is expected of you. But there is also a time for the ending of mourning when the clothes are discarded and life returns to normal. One of the difficulties of our stiff upper lip syndrome is that the process of grieving is not made easy by relatives or friends. People tolerate some show of emotion at the funeral, but are embarrassed by any later show of grief. Indeed, from then on we tend to act as if the dead person had never existed. He or she is never mentioned in the hearing of the bereaved person in case it should bring on any emotion. So not only do we have no stated time for grieving, but there is no end to the process, and most widows and widowers in English society become lonely and isolated for long periods after the death of their partner – some never recover.
    In much the same way many religions and nearly all primitive peoples, have a very definite start and end to the process of adolescence and the move into adulthood. In Western societies the process has neither a beginning nor

Releasing tensions

59

an end. Adolescence is a time of great emotional stress. One is learning what it is to be an adult, yet there is no induction into the state of adulthood. With increasing specialisation the student moves from the world of school to that of college, or employment – or sadly these days unemployment – without a recognised point at which he has achieved adult status. One might have a birthday card with a key on it, or a party at eighteen or twenty-one, but nothing really changes. Life would almost certainly be easier with an emotional and physical landmark when one accepts the full responsibilities of adult status and after which others recognise you for what you are – a fully-fledged adult with a place of your own within our society.

Stress due to factors in the individual

Temperament largely genetically determined

Everyone reacts differently to stress. Some like challenge and actively seek it in dangerous sports like hang-gliding or mountaineering. Others feel dizzy at the thought of going up in a chair-o-plane at the fair. Temperamentally, everyone is different. We are all individuals through our own unique blend of genes. Even identical twins are not exactly identical in their biochemistry, although they may look alike. As we all know, children in the same family are usually completely different in temperament. The differences are due to their genetic uniqueness and to their experiences in the family. Although we think we treat all our children alike, the fact is, we do not. For example, experience in the womb is different depending on the way the mother is living while she is carrying the child. The chemicals she takes into her body in food, drink and medicines affects them both as does her emotional state. The interaction between individuals in the family affects each differently and affects developing personalities. Our basic temperament is certainly largely genetic, but the developing personality of each child is conditioned by the way in which he or she is brought up in the family.

Personality largely socially determined

The family plays a most important part in the mental balance or imbalance of the individual. It moulds the personality, not by what is taught, but by the values, the attitudes and the beliefs evident in all relationships and behaviour which the child sees and experiences every day of its young life. Our attitude to pain, to distress, to the way in which we face a crisis or disaster, all are learned from

60

those around us in our youth. A happy, buoyant resilient attitude, one which sees every new experience as something pleasurable for interest and enjoyment, is perhaps the ideal preparation for coping with the later stresses of life.

This can only be engendered from a very early foundation of complete trust and confidence in not only the mother and father but also the other adults with whom the child comes in contact. Any insecurity in this early stage destroys the basis of trust and confidence and may have a lasting affect on the personality. To find out your own unique blend of personality types, and your reaction to stress, turn to page 000 and do your personality quiz.

*   *   *

So the reasons why there are high stress triggers in Britain today are only too plain to see. Society is in a state of flux, and it may take another generation to move through this period and find greater stability. We have to remember through these difficult times that we are the most adaptable of all the species on earth and the fact that we are all alive (although stressed) proves that we are adapting remarkably well to all the changes. For example, take that very small mobile family unit. It may sometimes find itself isolated, but, when you come to think about it, it is the ideal unit for today's industrial needs. Being small and mobile, it is able to upsticks and move to different locations with comparative ease. The old family network could never have done this.

Again, the changing roles of men and women mean that there are two wage earners in the family and a better standard of living can be achieved than was possible in the past. Also the change from the economically planned marriage of our forefathers to today's marriage for romantic love, means that there can be a real partnership between husband and wife, and this is now in the process of development. It is possible for a much stronger family bond of affection to develop with the father caring equally for the children and playing an active role in their development. This stronger family bond can make for greater emotional, economic and social support for all its members.

There are also answers to the rush hour, to traffic jams, and to pollution. Industry is being encouraged to move out of cities into the countryside. The New Towns, for example, are better planned and have more open space than the congested sprawls of the conurbations. We will undoubtedly witness a concerted move back into the countryside during the next decade. So take heart: we do control our own lives and most of us can decide where we are going to live. We can decide now what we want from life, and what we are going to do to achieve it.

CHAPTER 4

Who is particularly affected by stress today?

'Everyone,' I hear you say. And you are absolutely right. We all have our difficulties, problems and irritations. How stressed we allow ourselves to become, is governed by four main factors: our heredity, our upbringing, our personality and the environment we live in. A part of that environment is our work environment. This becomes particularly important in an industrial society because it gives us our place in that society. Some of us – because of our jobs, or lack of them; because of where we live, or with whom and among whom we live – are inevitably subjected to more stress triggers than others. Some of us – because of our personality – put high stressors upon ourselves, and thereby unknowingly lay ourselves open to heart disease, or other stress-induced illnesses. These are some of the problems with which we will be dealing in this chapter.

We will group these problems under the headings of physical stress, emotional stress, and social stress; and then follow with stress at work. The division into physical, emotional and social stress is, of course, an arbitrary one. The point of attempting to identify the main stress triggers like this is that different bio-chemicals are mobilised according to how emotionally stressed or physically stressed we are. Forewarned, they say, is forearmed and with a little knowledge we can take these stressors in our stride, and even enjoy outwitting them.

Let us first look at the reason for a great deal of stress in the community at present. In the Western world we are facing high stressors principally because we were the first in the industrial field. Our old industries are now slowing down and giving way to new ones. Coal is currently having to compete with oil as a major source of power just as oil will have to compete with nuclear power in another decade or

Workers in declining industries

63

so. Furthermore, new countries enter the industrialisation race and we now face fierce competition from countries in which we once had a monopoly of trade. This situation leads to high stressors among those brought up in the old industries and whose livelihood and way of life depends upon them. They are faced with redundancies and unemployment and the stressors are those of insecurity and fear of the future for themselves and their children.

The old industrial workforce

These are all affected by the changing industrial pattern. Many of the old mining pits, for example, are exhausted and have to be closed, while more are not economic to operate in the face of fierce competition from other countries. Many communities are tight-knit and the threat of alteration to the long-established way of life is a very high stressor for miners. Steel workers, ship builders and dockers also face redundancies and the loss of their previously highly-valued skills. Shipping, previously the main means of transport, is giving way to air, to the cross-channel ferries and the road juggernauts. The time is fast coming when change will be so rapid that one will have to acquire more than one skill in a lifetime and be prepared to work in different fields both here and abroad.

The unemployed

As other countries catch up in the technological race and go through their own industrial revolutions, the developed world – long the provider of goods for the underdeveloped – faces a major problem of unemployment. Every developed country now has a wholly unacceptable unemployment level, and in an industrial society unemployment is a major stress. It is not just a case of losing a wage packet, for redundancy payments have reduced the financial stress. The stress is social. You have lost your place in society, and a part of yourself. The part lost is the 'work self', the 'what you do in life', which in many ways is 'what you are'.

The loss of an occupation in an industrial society is a loss of part of yourself, and this is the reason why long-term unemployment, or retirement, is so stressful. Far too many working people do not live for much more than a year after retirement, which is due to the stress of loss. It is for many people a bereavement – a loss of the work self.

Redundancy, retirement or unemployment are factors which are usually imposed upon us by society. However there are other stressors that we impose upon ourselves, often unknowingly.

64

Those who stress themselves physically

The days when people were pushed beyond the limits of physical endurance have long since gone. We no longer use slave labour, kidnap men to man our ships, or subject prisoners to hard labour. Today, it is increasingly we ourselves, not an overseer or a boss, who subject our bodies to physical strain.

Long hours of hard training for sports, plus the strain of competition or performance can become just too much for the body to take, with the result that all normal functions gradually come to a halt while the body strives to put everything into meeting the special demands being put upon it. In women, this is clearly demonstrated when their monthly periods stop. This can happen, for example, in the condition known as Anorexia Nervosa when insufficient food is taken in to meet the work the body has to do, and something has to be sacrificed. But what I want to highlight here is a different condition. It is the deliberate policy of stressing our physical system so hard that it has to suspend its other normal work to meet the high energy needs demanded of it. Athletes, ballet dancers and some dedicated joggers come into this category.

Overtaxing the system

Research just completed on women joggers, who also play tennis and squash to 'keep fit', has shown that the cessation of periods is due to particular chemicals being released at the same time as the catecholamines – the stress chemicals. These chemicals (eg Met Enkephalon and Beta Endorphin) also give the 'high' which induces joggers to go on to ever greater efforts. Jogging for ten miles a day and playing tennis or squash is placing far too much physical strain on the body, and in most women, if this is done, their periods will cease. Exercise, if it is not to be a high physical stressor, needs careful control. It is essential to work with the pulse rate as a guide to the fitness of your heart and circulation. This has to be developed slowly. (See Chapter 11.)

Joggers

The typical Type A personality, the hard driving, striving individual who continually reacts with anger and irritation to every setback, is putting most strain on his heart and circulation. Such people punish the heart, particularly if they are the sort of people whose everyday pattern of reaction to minor setbacks is one of anger. (To see if you

The Type A personality

65

are a Type A personality do the test in the next chapter)

Heart strain   The public image of heart disease has got us all in a bit of a
state. We know that it is the highest cause of death in the
UK. We watch our comedians collapse on the stage, and
we are bombarded with warnings against 'risk factors' such
as heredity, high blood pressure and cholesterol. We are
warned off dairy produce, ('Don't eat butter', 'Don't eat
eggs',) told to cut down on meat, fat, salt, cigarettes,
alcohol; and so it goes on until it is small wonder that we
feel that everything we like in life is prohibited. It seems
that all the goodies are fattening, will silt up our arteries or
kill us off in our prime.

The fact is that our bodies need cholesterol and it is made
from the oils, glycerines and fatty acids in our diet. In
addition, we need plenty of fresh fruit, vegetables and
sufficient wheat and whole grain products to balance them.
More important still is regular exercise. The really vital
factors in beating heart disease are a job we enjoy, food
that has plenty of variety in it, plenty of walking to unfur
our arteries, adequate rest and sleep, people around us
whom we love and enjoy being with, more contentment
and happiness and less worry, anxiety, depression, irritation and anger.

The way the heart functions is closely related to effort.
Athletes who demand high effort from their hearts train by
gradually increasing its strength so that high effort is
achieved by a larger heart stroke instead of a faster beat.
Most of us, however, not only do not train the heart to
increase its strength but actually allow it to lose its normal
fitness. Then we take on a new job which demands continuous hard effort, and we drive hard by also playing
squash to keep ourselves 'fit'. What we are driving, however, is an engine with furred up pipes incapable of sustaining
in its present state the fast flow of energy we are demanding
from it. Then we find ourselves faced with angina, myocar-
dial infarction or a coronary.

So do not waste time worrying about butter, eggs and
milk. Concentrate instead on gradually developing a
strong heart. If you must be a strong driving type (although
we would rather you were not) control that anger pattern
of yours and do not despair. Then you could live to be a
hundred. Take your personality test, and if you prove to be
a Type A, then take your anger test. If you should rate
highly in this, then you should carry out the first aid
measures which you will find in Chapter 8.

Those who stress themselves emotionally

Developing technology can bring many benefits, it can also present us with many new problems. In the past, if serious malformations occurred during very early growth and development, nature endeavoured to remedy the situation and rarely allowed development to continue to birth. Today, medical science can save nearly all those who would not have previously survived, and so many more handicapped children are born. Mothers of these severely handicapped children have the high stress of guilt, particularly if they had taken any drugs in the early days of their pregnancy. Their fear is that in some way they are responsible for the child's condition. On top of this they have the added stress of the constant care of a helpless baby daily growing heavier and more difficult to cope with – and no end in sight. There is also the dreadful fear of what will happen to their child when they are no longer there to care. This is an ever increasing area of stress today but because the numbers are so large, organisations have sprung up to help relieve some parents for holidays while others provide care for longer periods of time. Helpful addresses will be found in Appendix 2.

Living with a handicapped child

It is no fun being an adolescent in our Western society. There are the uneasy swings of emotion as their biochemistry changes send them from alternate elation to depths of misery and tears. There is anxiety and fear for the future, the ridicule for those who try to stay 'pure', and the prestige in their own peer group for those who indulge in sexual exploits. For girls there is the added fear of pregnancy and the conflict of family, pill and family doctor to be resolved. Added to this, there is the constant pressure from home and school to do well and to achieve, often when contemporaries are already free and out in the adult world.

The problem of being a teenager

It is so much easier to pull the clothes over their head and to stay in bed, easier still to not wake up, or to drink to oblivion. All adolescents need a great deal of love and understanding and, above all, free and honest communication with the adults in their world. Support is all important at this very stressful time of life. If you find it difficult or impossible to talk to your teenagers yourself, find a friend of the family who can, and start to learn and understand their fears and anxieties. Alcohol consumption, drug taking and the suicide rate among teenagers is sadly on the increase.

One-parent families

The problem of adolescence is probably made very much more acute in cases where a single parent is trying to cope alone. In the last ten years the number of one-parent families has risen to over twelve per cent, or one in eight of all British families. The majority of their children under eight years of age have usually been given into the custody of the mother, but the sight of father alone pushing the pram, doing the shopping and looking after the children, is becoming more common as wives walk out of the home and custody is given to the father. The number of families headed by the man alone is now over 100,000, and the number of children who have to depend for their upbringing on father alone is in the region of 160,000.

The distorted home

The figures quoted above include the families of widows and widowers, but the vast majority of one-parent families result from breakdown or disruption. The stressors affecting the children appear to be variable. From research carried out on one-parent families, the stress of losing a parent by bereavement showed very little effect on the children's attainment and behaviour at school. They adjusted remarkably well. The stress of losing a father or mother by divorce appears to have more lasting effects. The child feels that he has been left deliberately, and in consequence feels rejected. One well-known researcher of the problems and stresses of children says that it is the 'distortion' of the family by divorce rather than the 'disruption' caused by bereavement, that is so detrimental to a child's development.

Those who stress themselves socially
Man is a gregarious creature. Like lions, we are meant to live in a social group and we need the support and companionship of our fellow men. This group acts as a reflection and gives us the knowledge of who and what we are vis-a-vis our society. Fat, thin, beautiful, ugly, talented, stupid – these words only assume meaning when there is a chance for comparisons. Loneliness, therefore, is a high social stressor as it affects our own self-support and our own self-knowledge.

This is a very much wider problem than one might imagine. *The extent of*
It affects all ages and stages of life. It is estimated from the *loneliness*
few surveys that have been carried out that as many as
three million people may be affected, including nearly half
of the single adult population and over a quarter of the
married population. If children were included the numbers
would be very much higher. Many of the elderly who are
unable to move about freely, and often unable to afford to
maintain their own transport, are very cut off from normal
social contact. Particularly hard hit are the naturally shy,
living in the country without the attraction of local shops to
bring them out of their homes. These people gradually
develop a house-bound pattern, and the rarer the social
contact the more withdrawn and isolated they become.
Even if they are married they tend to leave all the shopping, outdoor activities and socialising to their partners.

The young who leave home and travel to a city to live and *The lonely*
work are often badly affected by loneliness. All they can *young*
afford is a bed-sitting room and when their door is shut
there is nothing to take them outside to join in the life of
the rest of the house which they can hear going on around
them. Many will close the flat door on a Friday evening and
see no one and speak to no one until Monday morning.
Some of the loneliest children I have met are those in the
very large comprehensive schools. The distances between
classrooms on different floors and in different buildings are
vast and the children have to grab their books at the end of
one lesson and run to get to the next one in time. Being in
different groups for different subjects, they have little time
to find out even the names of others in the classes, and
there is no time to develop friendships.

There are those who have lost love, whether through *Who else is*
bereavement, separation, divorce or the ending of a love *lonely?*
affair. Love can also die in a marriage leaving either or
both partners tragically alone, though appearing compati-
ble in public. People with isolated jobs such as lighthouse
keepers or travelling salesmen can be lonely. So can own-
ers of small businesses whose work leaves no time for the
meeting or making of friends. And there are many more.
People who work unsociable hours. Single parents whose
commitments leave no time for socialising. Service and
company wives who are frequently on the move with their
husbands, and, above all, the shy. Also lonely are those

who have outlived their real friends, or who suffer reduced incomes and feel no longer able to keep up with their accustomed social commitments.

Loneliness is a high social stressor with a definite series of stages. At first there is insecurity and unease in relationships followed by the difficulty of making contact as unease increases. The third and last stage is the withdrawing from the painful effort and a life lived more and more in isolation. The stressors often start in childhood when the first images of ourselves are being formed. Children may be loved and wanted and feel worthy of a place in society, or they may be unloved, unwanted and feel rejected by separating parents. These images may be wholly false, but how many parents continually assure their children that they love them? Many of the more serious and intractable cases of anxiety, despair or depression have a background of double or treble rejection. First there is the disrupted home (children often feel that the parent who leaves the family has personally rejected them), then a possible rejection in one or more love affairs. The young person then feels unworthy of love and despairingly lonely. It is a stress situation akin to bereavement, but possibly longer lasting. Only the warmth of social contact and social support can right it.

CHAPTER 5

Work stress

There has been a great deal of research into work stress in Sweden, Canada and the United States, and now many other industrialised and industrialising countries are following suit. Let us first look at a composite of the research into work stress. The following areas have been found to be particularly stressful.

Imposed restraints	Noise, glare, unrealistic targets, high work overload or underload, unchosen teams, restricted movement.
Organisational factors	Lack of communication, no positive feedback on performance, no acceptance of new ideas.
Role in organisation	Lack of defined limits or authority, no definite role specification, inter-departmental conflicts, conflict with superiors, conflict with colleagues/staff, difficulty in delegation.
Relationships	Inability to get on with people.

How these potential stressors, which exist to a certain extent in all large organisations, affect the individuals working there, is due to the vulnerability of the individual at any one time. Vulnerability is governed by the following factors:

1 Our experience for the job.
2 The support of a group of colleagues at work.
3 The support of a caring home background.
4 The number and degree of stressors at any one time. (See Chapter 3, *How much change should you allow in your life?*)

71

5 Our personality. (See Chapter 6, *What kind of person am I?*)
6 Our present lifestyle. (See Chapter 10, *Lifestyle.*)
7 Our ability to cope with stress.

What sort of things do people find stressful?

What do you find most stressful in your job?
   'An unexpected visit from a director of the firm.'
What do you feel and how do you react to it?
   'Well, I try to appear confident but I'm on the defensive all the time. I'm apprehensive about the reason for the visit and can feel myself getting more and more tense. There's fear too. If our productivity figures aren't good we might be closed down. There's no real communication during the visit and you don't know how you stand or if your organisation is better or worse than the others. There's just fear and anxiety and this remains after the visit as you wait for any repercussions.'
What else do you find stressful?
   'Writing reports. Anger and irritation at having to do them in the first place and worry and anxiety that I am doing the right thing. What after all does Head Office want to know? There is no formula laid down, and there is never any feedback as you never know what you have written is well- or ill-received. This leads to some anger and frustration when the next one is due, so they tend to get shorter and shorter and my anxiety, frustration and anger get disproportionately larger.'

Some common stressors of managers
Lack of information

'Feeling angry at being kept in the dark and frustrated at not being able to communicate intelligently with my staff.'
Non-communication
'Feel "let them get on with it". But never let everything get into a mess. I'm aware of what is going on, but I never let the staff know I am annoyed. That would cause uproar.'
The pressure of time
'Not enough time to do any job to my satisfaction. My first reaction is "leave it". My second is to walk around my office and plan, and my third reaction is satisfaction at having done it to my own satisfaction.'
Unrealistic deadlines
'I get so angry at those people sitting up there planning things in their ivory towers. They know nothing of the problems, the staff shortages, the absence and illness rates,

72

the day-to-day running problems. My main stress is not being in control to resolve all these problems.'

Incompetent colleagues
'I get irritated, frustrated angry. I bang doors and desks and walk about the office to cool down. I feel like doing everything myself to make sure that it is properly done.'

Having to tell people they are not pulling their weight
'I feel very tense if I have to tell people off. I'm not very good with people. I was always very shy as a child, that's why I went in for chemistry – it's a non-people profession. Now I have landed up managing a factory. I would rather be in a laboratory by myself or with my technicians. I feel in charge there.'

Having to move to another area
'I get very depressed. Not for myself – I quite enjoy the prospect of being able to start again in a new location leaving present problems behind. No, it's having to tell my family. My wife hates moving. The house has to be sold just as she has got it right. The children get upset at having to leave their school and their friends. It creates untold problems for them. The gloom and disruption last for months.'

Staff shortages
'Dealing with overpressed staff and their stresses during holiday periods and through absenteeism when we are really short-staffed. Irritation and anger at budgets which don't permit adequate temporary arrangements. Anger at Head Office for not making exceptions due to our particular pressures. Frustration at not being able to do anything about it all.'

Do women experience more stressors just because they are women? Apparently they do and the most common ones are:

Different stressors of women managers

Being the first woman in a particular job
'The main feeling is one of isolation. There is no support, no one with whom to talk over the problems of the job. There seems to be almost a sort of men's club here, a kind of camaraderie which I'm conscious of not understanding. I feel an outsider.'

Having to stay alone in a hotel
'I hate having to go to the bar and dine alone. If I am tired I funk it and have sandwiches and coffee in my room, and then feel alone and stupid for having given in. I'm then

73

aware that I am not at my best at the following day's meeting. The men seem to manage better because they have already got matey at the bar.'

Being conspicuously different
'One feels exposed – almost like being in a goldfish bowl. Top management are just waiting for mistakes as they don't really expect a woman to be capable of doing a top job. Subordinates, especially women, are looking for signs of failure or weakness. One feels very vulnerable and I feel very tense.'

A felt lack of support
'Men have wives and families. Few of us have that sort of supportive background. We need a wife, a lover and a permanent escort. Society is not quite ready for us as a breed, and the stressors are high.'

There are a lot of other stressors too, such as:
– Lack of confidence in speaking in public.
– Diffidence in putting over a point of view.
– Inability to sustain a logical argument without getting emotionally involved in the outcome.
– Lack of confidence in their own ability to do the job really well.
– Inability to cope effectively with conflict in the organisation.

Workforce stressors

Lack of communication (retail store)
'Frustration. No one tells you what's going on. In the end you just give up and don't care. If they want to be like that, let them.'

Noise (canning factory)
'That's what is stressful. The noise is something dreadful. You can't hear yourself speak and it just goes on day after day and year after year with no let up. That's what kills you, noise.'

Time pressure (car assembly)
'Time is stressful. You have to clock yourself in and clock yourself out. It rules your life. The paced assembly doesn't stop and you have to keep up, no matter what you feel like. You can't slope off for a quick draw.'

Too many bosses (typist)
'Everyone runs you. It's drop this and do that. It's why are you doing that? That's not urgent – tell her I said so. You are like the jam in the sandwich, trying to please everyone and it's just impossible. I feel like chucking it all in.'

74

What do you find most stressful?

Do this quiz and find out your work stress score. They are fairly typical situations which everyone meets from time to time, and they should be taken in one's stride. However, if they occur frequently, you will have to take active steps to reduce their number, or improve your overall balance of health, and develop support groups outside your work to

	Never	Rarely	Sometimes	Often	Always
I cannot get my work finished in time.	1	2	3	4	5
I haven't the time to do things as I would like them to be done.	1	2	3	4	5
I'm not clear exactly what my responsibilities are.	1	2	3	4	5
I haven't enough to occupy my mind or my time.	1	2	3	4	5
Too many people make demands on me.	1	2	3	4	5
I don't get on with my boss.	1	2	3	4	5
I lack confidence in dealing with people.	1	2	3	4	5
I have unsettled conflicts with other staff.	1	2	3	4	5
I get very little support from my colleagues or my superiors.	1	2	3	4	5
I never know how I am getting on in my job. There is no feedback.	1	2	3	4	5
No one understands the needs of my department.	1	2	3	4	5
Our targets/budgets are unrealistic and unworkable.	1	2	3	4	5
I have to take work home to get it done.	1	2	3	4	5
I have to work at weekends to get everything done.	1	2	3	4	5
I can never take all my leave.	1	2	3	4	5
I avoid any difficult situations.	1	2	3	4	5
I feel frustrated.	1	2	3	4	5
Total score...........................					

enable you to cope with them. On the right you will see how often they occur – never, rarely, sometimes, often, and always. After each sentence ring the score that applies to you, and then add up your total.

How do you score?

0 – 20 The stressors are about average for most people who enjoy their work but inevitably find things frustrating from time to time.

21 – 45 The stressors are such that you get tense and uptight from time to time and you will need to follow the relaxation techniques in Part II.

45+ The stressors are too high. Are you perhaps a Type A personality, a worrier or a perfectionist? Do the Personality Test in Chapter 6 to find out if you are in a high-risk group for stress. If you are, follow the First Aid Programme given for your own personality type.

Shift work

Some people feel it to be stressful while others adapt to it easily. Adaptation depends upon many factors and one of these is where you live. In one area, almost everyone was employed by the Electricity Generating Board. Everyone worked shifts, so it was the social norm and all entertaining, parties and general get-togethers were planned around this pattern. There were very few problems. Another adaptation is where the whole family works a shift pattern and aims to work the same shifts. Again, socialising is planned around the timing of the shift work.

There are a lot of problems though and some of the usual ones are:

'I'm a single parent and it is very hard to get people to look after the children. With hours like mine, people are reluctant to help.'

'The problem is that everyone else works nine to five, Mondays to Fridays. All the social life is organised at weekends and you just can't join in, so you never make friends.'

'It's tough on the children. They like me to play football with them and take them to see the games. They don't understand why I have to go to bed in the daytime.'

'Shift work affects your sex life. It gets all upset. The night shift is the worst. It alters your personality and you become difficult to live with, and then there is divorce and living apart.'

'It's not me personally that suffers from rotating shifts – it's the family. I get moody and bad tempered on nights. I am short with the kids and we are all at loggerheads with one another.'

'Shift work has ruined my life. It could have been so good. It gave me extra money and time, and I built my own house and I thought I was happy doing that. But it wrecked my social life. My wife couldn't stand it and it wrecked our marriage. I have now built a yacht from a kit and I have got everything, but really I have got nothing. It's all to do with shift work.'

'People don't understand sleeping during the day. Dogs bark and motorists blow their horns and people play loud music. It's worst at the weekends in the summer. Motor mowers are going, children are shouting and yelling, and sometimes I don't sleep for three or four days at a time, then exhaustion takes over.'

'When you have leave and are away from shift work for a couple of months, then you begin to realise how jaded and lousy you feel most of the time. One month isn't long enough to get normal.'

'My health is poor on night shifts. I can't focus my eyes. They are getting very tired and painful. I get apathetic and slow too. I can't think and I can't say what I want to say. It takes me five or six days to recover from night shift.'

'You have got to have a car because public transport is geared to day workers. You get exhausted as the nights build up, and you don't sleep by day, and then you fall asleep at the wheel.'

'I think drink is the biggest problem. We all drink a lot. There is no social life, you work different hours to most people, so me and the boys on night shift have our own socialising and drink, that's all you can do.'

'No bosses see you and they don't know you. You do good work but it is the day people who get all the credit. It's very unrewarding.'

Whether or not shiftwork is stressful depends upon one's social supports as we have already seen, but it also depends upon the pattern of the shifts in comparison with our own time schedules – our biological clocks. We have many such clocks governing all our intricate bodily systems and balances. These are all affected by our own twenty-four-hour clock, which is actually just over twenty-four hours in most people. So the times for waking and sleeping, and the timing of the different waking activities such as fluid control, together with the timing of the sleeping activities such as tissue repair, are put out of their time phase if we try to impose another pattern on top of them. We do adapt slowly to continuous alteration, as when we move to another country, but there are people who never adapt, and it is questionable whether the waking/sleeping timescale itself ever adapts. The best solution is to have shifts organised in a pattern that progresses forwards to accord with our own twenty-four-hour plus cycle, and to give sufficient rest periods for people to catch up on their sleep loss.

Working hard:
three cases

We have heard of people working themselves into the ground and suddenly cracking up from stress. We have unions pressing for a five-day week and a six-hour day. So, are long hours of work bad for our health, or even lethal? Let us look at some of the patterns.

Jill is studying for her A-levels. She gets up at 6 am and puts in two hours work before school. After getting home from school she works till about 10 pm. She finds studying a slog, but it is going well. She is well supported by her family, and something is always planned for her for the weekends to get her out of the house.

Richard works a sixteen-hour day most days of the week. With going out to buy his own supplies, and having to do his own correspondence, estimates and accounts, he works practically seven days a week. He is pressed, often has difficulty in getting his money in, but is happier working for himself than he was when he had a steady job with a regular pay packet.

Kay is a housewife. She has four children of six, eight, eleven and thirteen years of age. Her husband is an accountant, a stickler for routine and always doing the 'right thing in the right way'. The two eldest children are beginning to rebel, and Kay tries desperately to keep the peace. She works a very long day getting up at 6 am to make all the

78

family's packed lunches and is often getting the children's school clothes ready at ten at night. Her husband cannot understand why these things are not done 'at the proper time'. She grows nearly all their fruit and vegetables, makes most of their clothes, and is on Valium (unbeknown to the family) for her 'nerves'.

These three all work long hours, but Kay is the only one who suffers from high stressors. Theoretically, she is the only one who could sit down and relax, but she never does. Jill's and Richard's efforts are something they want to do, and the result for them is real satisfaction. Kay's effort is imposed upon her, and the result for her is distress. That inevitably includes anxiety and depression, which are discussed in Chapters 13 and 14.

PART II

Stressmanship in action

In this part of the book, we really get down to the business of what to do about stress in our lives. We have called it *Stressmanship in Action* because there is no single approach which we could identify with a title like handling, coping with, or even managing stress. There are, in fact, a number of approaches which include:

1 Stress Reduction – dampening down the automatic response when not needed.
2 Stress Arousal – actively calling on Adrenalin when needed.
3 Pre-stressing – training to meet stress.
4 Stress Proofing – Developing resilience through a healthy life style.
We will be concerned mainly with stress reduction and stress proofing.

Dampening down is needed when the heart rate and blood pressure rise but there is no outlet for activity, such as when you are sitting at your desk, being hauled over the coals or sitting fuming in a traffic jam. Methods for stress reduction will be found in Chapter 8.

Stress reduction

This is the active use of the stress response when you need it, for example, to stay awake to complete an emergency task. This will switch on as you increase your motivation for a particular task.

Stress arousal

This is the art, which should begin in early childhood, of

Pre-stressing

learning to meet the small everyday stressors of life in order to develop resilience. It is also definite training to be able to meet regular anticipated stressors such as the problems of having to police an antagonistic area or having to live with the continuous threat and violence.

Stress proofing   The development of a lifestyle that raises one's resistance to high pressure and safeguards one from heart disease, hypertension and all the other stress-induced diseases. (See Chapter 10.)

So you see, there is not just one way of meeting stress. There is handling it and coping with it when it occurs, there is the active summoning up of it when it is needed, and there is the raising of our resistance so that we can tolerate it.

One of the major parts of Stressmanship is knowing how we react to, and interact with, stress. Why, for example, do some of us seek it in sport for the thrill of danger? Why do others demand a highly stimulating atmosphere at work and stress everyone around them? Why do some of us shun every form of difficulty and problem and run away from them, while others can only be creative in the midst of noise and turbulence? We are, of course, all different, with different personalities, needs, anxieties, hopes and fears. One overall approach could never be effective for so many diverse types. The first essential therefore is a clear understanding of the type of person that *you* are.

Some of what you are is hereditary, while some is a mixture of heredity and environment, and some other parts, such as language, are developed in social interaction with other people, particularly your family. Early experiences before the age of six or seven are vital in the formation of personality, and these experiences will affect a great part of your behaviour and needs today. So the foundation chapter of Stressmanship in Action, *What kind of person am I?* is all about you and how you became what you are.

CHAPTER 6

What kind of person am I?

The kind of person you are now is the sum total of many different things, some inherited and some developed in social interaction in one's own environment, as the following shows:

The Parts of Personality

Social and environmental:	The self concept – the 'Who I am' as known to oneself
Inherited but developed socially:	Temperament and intelligence
Inherited:	Body build and physiological constitution

All of these are part and parcel of our personalities. Temperament and intelligence are largely inherited, but the kind of intelligence, like thinking logically and speaking a particular language, only develop when we are with other people, so that it is part genetic and part socially developed. The self concept, 'who I think I am', is developed first in the family and then in the wider society of school, friends and work. The interaction of our genetic inheritance and our social environment starts almost immediately, in fact in the mother's womb. This is really the developing baby's first social environment, and it has an effect on later behaviour. For example, a mother who is very tense and nervous throughout pregnancy will give birth to a tense and fretful child, because changes in the biochemistry of the mother react on the baby. It is essential to use calming stress reduction techniques (see Chapter 8) if you are going through a difficult and stressful period while carrying, because you will need a calm placid baby who will sleep at nights and allow you to do the same.

Our social selves   We will start with our social selves. What we think we are is learned from our earliest days, starting even before we can talk. We listen and hear the things that are said about us, and we take them in as being what we really are.

'I am' from the Family

I'm heavy.	I'm as light as a feather.
I have my father's nose (he was a great man).	I'm the image of my grandmother (No one in the family likes her).
I talk too much.	I'm shy.
I'm messy.	I'm always careful with my toys.
I'm not very bright.	I'm very good at maths.

'I am' from School

I'm good at games and sport.	I'm a duffer at games.
I'm a dunce at maths.	I'm quite bright if I try.
I can't spell.	I'm a fast reader.
I'm popular.	I'm not very popular.

Adult experiences   These either consolidate the above beliefs, or give a second chance, as it were, to appraise ourselves through the eyes of others.

Trusting the world   The most important event in our early years of life is the development of a sense of trust in this new environment outside the womb, and trust in the adults in our world. If this does not develop, the opposite trait – mistrust – does. Consistency, the sameness of experience, people reacting in the same way to the things we say and do, all give confidence that life and people are predictable and reliable. With trust comes the confidence to explore one's surroundings, relying on everything being friendly. Thus one develops confidence and friendliness – the opposite of aggression and hate. If there is discord in the family engendering fear or mistrust in the child, the personality cannot develop its full potential.

How we develop   The full developmental pattern of the parts of the personality such as basic trust, complete with their opposite de-

84

velopment, is given below together with the times of their development:

Birth to eighteen months
   Basic trust versus mistrust and fear of people.

Eighteen Months to three years
   Independence versus shame and doubt in one's abilities.

Three to five years
   Initiative and cooperation versus guilt and aggressive reactions.

Five years to puberty
   Industry and love of finding out versus inferiority and hanging back.

Adolescence
   Identity and 'I know who I am' versus confusion and search for 'what am I?'

Early adulthood
   Intimacy versus isolation and inability to make close relationships

Young adult
   Creativity and productivity versus stagnation.

Maturity
   Ego integrity versus despair.

The three to five year period, initiative versus guilt, is crucial for the development of cooperation with people instead of aggression and feelings of violence against them. Confirmation that aggression, as a general pattern of behaviour towards others, arises at this stage, comes from a study carried out in nursery schools. The childrens' scores of aggression were obtained from tests carried out at school and then visits were made to each home to assess each child's pattern of child rearing. The patterns which corresponded most highly with non-cooperative and aggressive behaviour in the child, were friction and discord in the home.

The seeds of aggression

	Agreement with child's aggression score
Friction over discipline of child	+ 57
Discord in the home	+ 41
Close relationship with child	− 61
Understanding of child's problems	− 59
Quickness of approval or disapproval of conduct	− 56
Democracy in child-rearing policy	− 52

You can see clearly how experiences with our fellow men, particularly with our families, either enhances our basic temperament and fulfils our needs, or stunts our social growth which may affect our personality for years.

Intelligence Intelligence is one of the components of personality which is of concern to parents, teachers, students and children alike. It can cause a great deal of distress, so we should say something about it here. Everyone seems to be concerned with peoples' IQ. How intelligent is my child? The significant question should be, what kind of intelligence has my child? You see, there is not just one kind of intelligence. There is verbal (language), numerical (number intelligence), spatial (the putting of things into relationship with each other), and mechanical intelligences plus abilities such as dexterity, reasoning, problem-solving (being able to put a car together) and so on. At best, IQ is only a very clumsy sampling technique. In the Western industrialised world, the prized intelligences are verbal, numerical and problem-solving. We rate both spatial and mechanical intelligence very low. Yet these are equally important skills.

Physiology is a term which covers the whole working of the brain (with its emotional centres) and the body, so we are really talking about the very foundations of your behaviour and the very basis of your personality. An important part of these are our defence systems, in particular (for us) our immunity to the stress-induced illnesses. We all differ in our immunity to, and our susceptibility to, allergies and to illnesses of all kinds. For example, all of your colleagues can have exactly the same diet in the canteen, yet one of you could develop a deficiency disease. Conversely, nearly everyone in an area could go down with 'flu during an epidemic, and one of you escape. We all differ in our resistance. However, we can all increase our resistance to illness (and thus stress) by the development of a healthy lifestyle, just as we can weaken it by a damaging lifestyle. (See Chapter 10.)

Your physiological constitution

If you are tall and thin, are you also happy-go-lucky and carefree with a laughing, jolly personality? The two do not really go together, do they? If you are tall and slender, you are probably also thoughtful and conscientious. It has always been recognised that a certain temperament goes with a particular body build. In Shakespeare's *Julius Caesar*, for example, we read that he needs people around him who are fat and amiable and who sleep at night. He distrusted Cassius, you remember, with his 'lean and hungry look' – he 'thinks too much'. Most screen professors are portrayed as what we call cerebral and linear types: very tall and thin. An American, Sheldon, has identified three types of body build related to the three layers of primary cells in the developing child. After the sperm has fertilised the ovum, the cells having rested begin to multiply until a large cluster forms. Inside this cluster, three distinct layers of cells develop – the outer, middle and inner layers which each form a particular part of body and brain.

Body build and temperament

The inner layer, the ENDODERM, forms our inner organs.

The middle layer, the MESODERM, forms our skeletal bones and our muscles.

The outer layer, the ECTODERM, forms the skin and coverings, including the brain.

Sheldon then describes his body types as:

ENDOMORPH with large body cavities and stomach: The rounded type.

MESOMORPH with muscular frame and square shoulders: The athletic type.

ECTOMORPH with long lean frame and small body cavities: The linear type.

**The relationship between
body build and temperature**

Endomorph
Rounded, relaxed, amiable, loves food and socialising, complacent, sleeps deeply and needs people when troubled.

Mesomorph
Loves physical adventure, energetic, needs exercise, likes to dominate, has a direct manner, has courage and needs action when in trouble.

Ectomorph
Over-intense, anxious, secretive, inhibited, sleeps poorly, introverted, restrained in posture and movement, needs solitude when troubled.

There is a great deal of research linking, with some success, different types of illness to these different kinds of body build. A score of 7 is given for each complete type. Few people are 7–1–1, (pure Endomorph) or 1–7–1, (pure Mesomorph) or even 1–1–7, (pure Ectomorph). Many are an average of, for example, 4–5–4 and some have been perfect mixes of 4–4–4. You are probably a mixture with a leaning to one or other basic build.

A Personality Test follows. This is designed specifically to identify your vulnerability to stress.

The Personality Test

Read through the description of each of the following sixteen situations, and choose the answer that you think *most nearly matches* what you would do. One cannot, of course, be exact as all situations depend upon the circumstances. So it is the nearest match. You may find it easier to eliminate as there are some things you certainly would not do. Score 3 for the chosen answer. If there is another answer that would be your second choice, score 2. Score your third choice 1.

So for most of the sixteen situations you will have three separate scores. If there is just one definite way in which you would react, and the rest certainly do not apply, then leave it at that one. We are nearly all a mix of personalities, and the reason for three scores in each situation is to indicate the mixture and the proportions in your case.

To minimise the extent to which your conscious or unconscious desire to be any particular type might influence your answers, the questions are given reference letters at random.

1 Something happens that throws out your plans for the day completely. Do you:

U   Worry about how to fit in the work which was planned?

V   Fume? You had a well-organised day planned and you hate having to throw it all to one side. You think out ways to keep some semblance of your planned day intact.

W   Bemoan the fact to all and sundry to enlist their sympathy?

X   Think philosophically, 'Well I suppose it could have been worse' and then see if you cannot pull some of the threads together and carry on?

Y   Find yourself glad to have a free day to plan something you had had in mind for some time?

Z   Feel angry and try to control it? You may pace up and down or bang a desk top in exasperation and then put all your energy into completely replanning the day.

2 You have a new boss who lets it be known that he does not approve of daytime drinking. Do you:

Z   Check with your colleagues to see what the general reaction is?

U   Think that it is an imposition and rig up a drinks

89

cupboard in a filing cabinet for yourself and your friends, but keep it dark?

V   Fail to make up your mind exactly what to do about it because you do like a drink at lunchtime but worry about the consequences of being thought a drinker in this new regime?

W   Think that the sociability at lunchtime may suffer a little but you will settle for orange or tomato juice and get your vitamins in? It's an ill wind that does not blow somebody some good. You will still meet in the bar.

X   Think it quite a good idea for the firm as one needs a clear head? You quite often have mineral water yourself at lunch.

Y   See no good reason to change now as you always have had a lager with your lunch each day?

3 A bus Inspector asks for your ticket. You have mislaid it and do not have sufficient money with you to pay again. The Inspector orders you off the bus. Do you:

Y   Hurriedly leave as you cannot stand scenes? You worry about the loss and whether you have lost anything else. You go over every move you have made from buying your ticket until now.

Z   Feel a little uncomfortable, apologise, and tell him you intend to pay, and give him your name and address?

U   Coolly take his number, say that you resent his manner and that you will be reporting him as you are sure that the Company's policy is not to order people off their buses if they are willing to furnish evidence of their identity?

V   Feel thoroughly put out with yourself? You have a particular place for your ticket and cannot understand why it is not there. You refuse to move.

W   Feel highly embarrassed and get off the bus as quickly as possible hoping that there was no one there who recognised you.

X   React with irritation that you could have been thought to have been taking a free ride? You give your name and address and stay firmly, and angrily, put.

4 You are offered a job some distance away with better pay and prospects. If you accept, it means leaving your numerous local activities through which you have made

many friends. Do you:

X   Remain unsure? The job may be difficult but you could do with that extra pay. You could move and find activities near the new job, but that might present problems.

Y   Decline? You are quite happy as you are and see no point in changing.

Z   Accept for the prospects which you take to mean quicker promotion? You have no fears about making new friends.

U   Dislike the idea of change? You have a good working routine and you would have to think about it very carefully. You do not like your way of life upset.

V   Decline? You would certainly like more money and promotion, but it would mean losing all your friends and your local activities.

W   Assess the job and its prospects first? Then assess the area and its facilities. Then come to a decision.

5 You have checked your football coupon and to your utter delight and astonishment it appears that you have won a very large sum of money. You tell your family in great delight only to find that the letter was not posted. Do you:

W   Burn inside and blame yourself for having given it to others to post? You know you should not have altered your regular pattern of posting. You shut yourself away and get depressed. Nothing in life goes right.

X   Explode and rant and rage at everyone in sight and then storm out?

Y   Become very depressed? You had worked out that the overdraft and the mortgage could now be paid off, but now your problems appear worse and less manageable than before.

Z   Console yourself and the family that you really do not need that new car you had been planning for, and arrange something to take all their minds off the disappointment?

U   Ring up all your friends with the story so that by the end of the evening you have got it all off your chest? If they were all out you think of getting quietly drunk and stay miserable.

V   Find out why it did not get posted and whose fault it was? Then make quite certain that it cannot happen again by making specific arrangements for posting in future.

6 A member of your group has been hauled over the coals for something he did not do. This may affect his future promotion prospects (and enhance yours). Do you:

V   Believe that it is a storm in a teacup and will blow over with no harm done?

W   Assess the situation thoroughly before doing anything?

X   Become involved in the case and befriend your colleague?

Y   Regard it as no concern of yours. You are sorry, of course, but you get on with your job?

Z   Immediately set about putting the record straight?

U   Wonder if there will now be a shake-up in your department as a result of this incident? You decide to look into your own records and files very carefully.

7 You have accepted a new job and it quickly becomes apparent that its scope and your responsibilities are far from clear. Do you:

Z   Go and talk it over with your immediate senior after taking the advice of your colleagues?

Y   Re-read the job specification carefully, note where the gaps are and ask for it to be clarified in writing?

X   Study the needs of the job, then map out the areas and limits and work to these, finally writing the job specification yourself?

W   Worry about what your responsibilities really are? If you ask for them to be clarified you may be thought an idiot for not knowing, and it might make the situation more difficult.

V   Get irritated with the lack of information and go and see the boss to hammer out a proper specification?

U   Work cheerfully within the obvious limits and the leave it at that?

8 There is a long queue at the supermarket checkout and someone wishes to pay by cheque and cannot find her cheque card. Do you:

Y   Relax and think pleasant thoughts while you wait more or less patiently?

X   Wonder why people cannot write their cheques in advance and organise their cheque cards in a holder so that they always know where they are?

W   Suddenly wonder if you have got your own wallet and purse and hurriedly check that they are there?

V   Find a supervisor and suggest that others could be dealt with while the customer searches for her card at leisure? You point out that some customers may be in a hurry.

U   Stand on one foot and then the other – getting more and more furious by the minute – and keep watching the time?

Z   Look around sympathetically and engage the nearest person in conversation?

9 Friends have entered you for a television programme that gets its laughs at the participants' expense. What is your reaction?

X   You are anxious that something unpleasant might happen to you like custard being poured over your head or a pie pushed in your face. No, you do not think you will go.

W   Astonishment. You certainly have not the time for that sort of thing.

V   Amused. You have seen the show and find it very funny. You are quite pleased they thought of you, but you do not accept.

U   Work out if the publicity would be good for you at this stage of your career.

Z   Certainly not. You think that these shows are childish and an intrusion into other peoples' privacy.

Y   You would not do it if it means going with total strangers. You might go with a good friend though.

10 You have just acquired your dream house. You are offered promotion which entails moving to a new area. What are your first thoughts?

W   You feel annoyed as you have everything settled, but accept if you feel you have to.

V   You will decline the offer and stay put.

U   You will find out if there are any people you know there before deciding.

Z   Accept the promotion and then go to the area and find a suitable property.

Y   Seek an early interview to find out the job specification and the prospects and then assess the situation objectively.

X   You worry about all the problems involved: the move to another house, the new responsibilities.

11 Your local charity is organising a parachute jump for which there will be some training. You are invited to take part. What is your reaction?

V   No. Why can they not do what they have always done? It always produced a good response.

U   There is very little training. There is so much that could go wrong. You think it is too risky.

Z   You would go along to see if there is some organisational job you could do to help.

Y   You have never jumped before, but will certainly have a go.

X   You had better find out first who else is going to train for the jump.

W   You are perfectly content with two feet on the ground, but you would go along to cheer them on.

12 A friend rings up to tell you that you have been chosen as a member of a team to visit China for a cultural exhange. Do you:

U   Feel uncertain if you will accept? It will mean being away when you have other commitments.

Z   Feel pleased, but apprehensive that the journey may be difficult and the language incomprehensible? And what about the risk of disease?

Y   Start thinking of the contacts you could make while you are there and ring up friends and acquaintances who might help with introductions?

X   Enthusiastically start planning the tour and find out the temperatures, the need for injections and visas, etc?

W   Ring around and try to find out who else is going and what they are planning to take?

V   Thank them for thinking of you and then get on with what you were doing when the call came?

13 You arrive at the station to find that your usual train is cancelled and that there is an hour's delay. Do you:

X   Buy a paper and settle down to read?

U   Look around and see what everyone else is doing, sympathise with them and wait as patiently as possible?

Y   Worry at the long wait? Think of all the things that are piling up and try to telephone the office? Find it difficult to settle down to read?

94

V   Feel mad at having your day disrupted, but you do not show it? You try and get on with the papers in your case, but nonetheless feel put out.

Z   Get irritated? You cannot tolerate the idea of wasting an hour on a platform. You go and find alternative transport or go for a walk round the town.

W   Get out your diary and see what has to be rearranged? Telephone and reorganise the morning. You decide to make up the lost time at the end of the day.

14 There is an accident practically blocking the middle of the road. There are many onlookers, but nobody seems to be doing anything. Do you:

Z   Go and talk to and console the injured?

W   Immediately get everyone organised to assist you in getting the traffic moving?

X   Drive around it feeling that these things are best left to the professionals?

U   Willingly join in to do what you can?

Y   Go to the nearest telephone, report the accident and then go on as you have a tight schedule?

V   You find accidents worrying and alarming and, feeling that you would be more of a hindrance than a help, drive on with a guilty feeling?

15 You have been offered a job with higher status but initially you would lose money because the allowances and perks that you have previously had do not accompany this promotion. Do you:

x   Find out who your boss would be and who you would be working with, and then if you like the people decide that you will accept?

V   Consider your position very carefully? It may be that for your career prospects, it is time to seek wider experience elsewhere. If so you accept.

Y   Feel that you are happy as you are, and as the family agree with you, there seems no point in changing your job?

W   Accept, believing that the rise in status is worth the drop in immediate income?

Z   Consider that it would mean more work and longer hours and you have your life well organised around your garden, your collections and your hobbies. You do not want to change things and you turn it down.

U   Wonder if you can handle it as it is a job with much

more responsibility? You decide to find out as much as you can about it first, consider whether you could manage on less money, and then decide.

16 Holidays and weekend breaks. What is your attitude towards them?

Y   I never take weekend breaks but I always take a full, annual holiday.

U   I like occasional weekend breaks in order to prepare for a particularly high work load. I always take all my holiday entitlement, but I still keep a close watch on what is going on.

Z   I do not think I have ever had all my leave. When I do take some, I never go away for the full period, there is so much to do at home.

V   I have not the time to take weekend breaks and I do not think I have had all my leave entitlement for years. If I do take a holiday I usually get right away to somewhere new and interesting.

X   I take all the breaks and holidays I can and relax completely. When I am away, I do not give work a thought.

W   I usually take all my holidays unless someone else is very pushed. I have stood in and helped others out from time to time.

Your Score
Card
Now transfer the scores you have already marked to the following score card. For each question in turn, take the scores 1, 2 or 3 and enter them in the line for that question in the score card, making sure that each score corresponds with the letter. For example, if you have scored to question 5, Z 3, Y 2 and V 1, then you would fill in line 5 on the card as follows:

     5. X( ) V(1) Y(2) W( ) Z(3) U( )

Question

1	Z( )	Y( )	U(3)	V(1)	X(2)	W( )
2	U( )	X(2)	V( )	Y(3)	W( )	Z(1)
3	X(3)	U(2)	Y(1)	V( )	X( )	W( )
4	Z( )	W( )	X(1)	U( )	Y(3)	V(2)
5	X(3)	V( )	Y(2)	W( )	Z( )	U(1)
6	W(3)	Z(2)	U(1)	Y( )	V( )	X( )
7	V( )	X( )	W(1)	Y(2)	U( )	Z(3)
8	U(3)	V( )	W(2)	X( )	Y( )	Z(1)
9	W( )	U( )	X(3)	Z( )	V(2)	Y(1)
10	Z( )	Y( )	X(2)	W( )	V(3)	U( )
11	Y( )	Z( )	U(2)	V(1)	W(3)	X( )
12	X(2)	Y( )	Z( )	U(3)	V( )	W(1)
13	Z( )	W(2)	Y(1)	V(3)	X( )	U( )
14	W( )	Y( )	V( )	X( )	U(3)	Z(2)
15	W( )	V(3)	U( )	Z(2)	Y( )	X( )
16	V( )	U(2)	Z( )	Y( )	X(3)	W(1)

Totals	( )	( )	( )	( )	( )	( )
Column	1	2	3	4	5	6

Now add up the marks in the first column entering the total in the brackets above the figure 1. Do the same in the other columns. The highest mark will be your predominant personality type and the other totals will give you your mix. Let us say that your score is:

(12)	(34)	(6)	(4)	(16)	(3)
1	2	3	4	5	6

Your predominant personality will be a definite No.2. and your mixture of personalities will be roughly half No.2. and a quarter No.1. and a quarter No.5. Now you will want to know what the numbers stand for.

Personality types		
Column	Type	
1	ATHLETIC:	hot ambitious
2	ATHLETIC:	cool dominant
3	LINEAR:	anxious worrier
4	LINEAR:	strictly precise
5	LATERAL:	easy going
6	LATERAL:	socially dependent

If your score for any of these is 33 or over, your personality is mainly that type which fashions your behaviour most of

97

the time. The degree of stress risk associated with each
type is:

The stress risk

Predominant personality type	Stress risk	Possible type of illness
1 Hot ambitious	High	Physical illness
2 Cool dominant	Low	Physical illness
3 Anxious worrier	High	Nervous system and physical illness
4 Strictly precise	Moderate	Nervous system
5 Easy going	Low	Physical illness
6 Socially dependent	Moderate	Nervous system

If you are a high risk personality, you should read all of the
next chapter to find out what your risks are, why they exist,
and what to do about them.

If you are a moderate risk personality, turn to page 106
in the next chapter.

If you are a low risk personality, move on to Chapter 9.

CHAPTER 7

Personality types and their stress risk

Personality types with a high stress risk.
These are the hot ambitious and the anxious worrier.

You are the worrier par excellence. You have marvellous qualities of conscientiousness and insistence on seeing that a job is well done, but you worry about every aspect of it. Worry is a good and useful attribute if it leads to an attack upon the problem. If it is just a state of worry without leading to any positive action, it is bad. The strain for you is obviously on the nervous system. So, if your defence systems are overwhelmed, any illness is more likely to be a panic attack or an anxiety state rather than a physical illness. It is essential that you learn how to relax, particularly the mind, to stop the problems going round and round without achieving either solution or resolution. The most helpful technique for you to master is the Relaxator Technique prepared especially for your personality type. From time to time you may well become depressed as anxiety and depression often follow one another. So after mastering the relaxation techniques in the next Chapter, move on to Chapters 13 and 14, *Depression* and *Anxiety*, and only after this, tackle the lifestyle, food and exercise chapters. Anxiety can be controlled with Relaxator Technique and the calming breathing at night when you go to bed will help to keep the worries from circling round in the mind, and help you to sleep soundly. Move on now to Chapter 8.

The anxious worrier

If this is your predominant type, you get yourself into a state of strain where the defence and immunity systems are weakened and over-burdened. The most likely consequential illnesses are hypertension (high blood pressure) or coronary heart disease. These arise from the continual 'anger and irritation reaction' to difficulties. Anger in-

The hot ambitious

99

creases the output of a particular biochemical – Nor Adrenalin – which stimulates the heart and circulation to give you the fighting pattern which your body chemistry senses that you need. This chemical process inside you has no means of knowing that you are not just about to start a sword fight, but are only sitting still and fuming which, as you and your types need action when troubled, only serves to increase your frustration, which in turn puts your blood pressure up even higher. So for you the most urgent thing to do is to handle the anger and irritation. First we have to

Test your anger and irritation pattern

		Never	Seldom	Sometimes	Usually	Always
1	I get irritated if I am kept waiting.	1	2	3	4	5
2	I get very irritated when other people slow me down at work.	1	2	3	4	5
3	I get really angry when people cannot think things out for themselves and keep running to me with every little problem.	1	2	3	4	5
4	I get angry when people continually interrupt me when I am busy.	1	2	3	4	5
5	I get annoyed when others do not appreciate my true worth.	1	2	3	4	5
6	I feel annoyed with myself when I make mistakes.	1	2	3	4	5
7	I cannot stand being laughed at. I get mad.	1	2	3	4	5
8	If things go wrong at home I usually feel irritation.	1	2	3	4	5
9	I get short tempered when the children do not behave themselves.	1	2	3	4	5
10	I get cross when people make stupid mistakes.	1	2	3	4	5
11	When people let me down I get really angry.	1	2	3	4	5
12	I feel that most problems or difficulties at work are due to other people's silly mistakes and that makes me angry. It's such a waste of time.	1	2	3	4	5

find out how serious the problem is for you, so do the following Anger Test by putting a ring round the figure that most truthfully answers each question, and then adding up your total score.

A score of up to 12 Are you sure? Try it again. No, I really do not believe it. You are not a true hot ambitious.

A score of 12–24 Not bad at all, though the pattern is starting. You were probably not a very hot ambitious early on in life, but the type is now in the making due to your particular work or circumstances. Reduce the striving pattern now by reading the next few chapters very carefully and start to practice the First Aid Techniques in the next chapter.

A score of 25–36 You have a fairly well-established anger pattern now, particularly if your score is above 30. It is likely that you sit fuming in traffic jams and in all the situations where you feel that you are not in full control or are at the mercy of other idiots. You must take stock now as you can not let this go on further without risking damage to your health. Begin by reading the next chapter, start to practice the stress reduction techniques and then move to Chapter 11, *Activity*, and begin to increase your resistance to heart and circulation problems.

A score of 37–48 This is high and you are running a considerable risk of hypertension (high blood pressure). I would suggest that you go to your own doctor and ask him check your blood pressure. Do not worry if it is slightly raised, you can bring it down with the stress reducing techniques described in the next chapter. Practice them, and carry them out faithfully, and you will reduce the pressure. Then read *Handling anger and irritation* which follows.

A score of 49 – 60 This is far too high, and is dangerous. These are the dangers for you:
1   Allowing the constant reaction of anger to raise your blood pressure also increases the production of the particular chemical Nor Adrenalin which stimulates the heart and pushes the blood pressure up higher in preparation for fighting. Unfortunately, our bodies do not know that we are not about to start a physical fight.
2   Cholesterol is being pushed out into the system to give you extra energy. This can attach itself to slack artery walls

and cause a clot and a blockage (*Thrombus* – hence coronary thrombosis – a clot in the circulation in the heart).

3 Playing highly competitive sports, such as squash, on top of a highly competitive occupation, puts additional strain on a heart already working overtime through the high anger pattern.

4 Allowing yourself insufficient time to relax properly, calm down the whole system and get back to normal.

5 Giving no time to non-competitive exercise like brisk walking in the open air, or swimming. These tone up all the muscles and the circulation without strain and relax the emotional system at the same time.

6 A high intake of alcohol (it often goes with your personality type) which puts more strain on the blood circulation.

As you read the above it will become clear how and why you really have to stop, right now, this heady rush to a coronary. Stop all competitive games for the time being, and walk or swim for your exercise. Go to your doctor and ask for a reading of your blood pressure, If it is up, do not worry as you can bring it down through the practice of relaxation techniques. Next learn and practice the First Aid techniques in the following chapter, especially the calming breathing which you should use whenever you feel the irritation and the anger rising. Now you will need some helpful ideas for trying to control the constant anger or irritation reaction which is damaging your heart. So we will try and tackle that next.

You can control anger and irritation successfully

You can control anger and suppress it, prevent it from rising, or let out the steam in the same way as one releases the valve on a pressure cooker. Controlling anger sounds effective, and indeed it is, but it has its very real drawbacks. Suppressed anger is still an anger pattern in the system and it has an effect on the lining of the stomach. The lining goes white in rage and the normal blood vessels are restricted. This affects its normal function of digesting food and you become prone to stomach upsets and gastritis, and may eventually end up with a gastric ulcer. So the suppression of anger is not a good idea. Preventing it from rising in the first place is the best remedy and there are techniques for this which we will go into later. However, there is the difficulty that if you have developed this very high irritable reaction to problems, your reaction will be too quick to

102

allow you to apply preventative techniques. So we have to attempt a release – 'letting off steam' first – which will gradually lead to a calmer you. This will take the strain off the heart and the blood vessels, and as this begins to take effect, the hot ambitious you will gradually become the cool ambitious.

The anger release pattern is not without difficulties. While we want release, we do not want it released by means of aggression towards people. So the whole object of anger release is that the method must be drawn away from people and directed at the inanimate environment, or to an inanimate object. If an object is chosen it has to be stronger and tougher than the individual, in order to avoid a link between anger release and destructive tendencies. There are so many different and efficient ways of anger release that I think the best thing to do is to recite them briefly after which you can select those that are most effective for you, and which suit your kind of life. *Anger release*

1 Leave the office or room, take a deep breath, get into an empty lift and yell, 'I hate everyone'; take a deep steadying breath and with a feeling of, 'Now I feel better and ready to love my fellow men again', come out of the lift, walk calmly down the stairs and restart life again. You can do the same in the rest room, the lavatory or an empty office. *Immediate release of anger*
2 Walk briskly in the open air, round the block, round the garden or the roof (if flat). Stop and look at something that takes your interest. Feel that life really has a lot to offer, drink it in and rejoin it.
3 Release the energy in constructive ways. This is often the best way if you are at home. Clean the windows (if you have not too much of a hate on, otherwise you might be tempted to smash them), scrub, polish, or anything that needs energetic application. Then stand back and admire what you have done. The linking of pleasure with anger release is important for restoring calmness and contentment, and if it is made standard practice after an outburst, it will help to control the anger pattern.
4 Link the energy release with something you enjoy or like after you have done it, like cleaning the car, renovating furniture, or doing any job that you have been wanting to do for some time. This will give you pleasure and turn the anger to good advantage making you feel happy about it. This positive after-effect is important.

I hope these will have given you a number of ideas. The main things to aim for are:

First, release of the anger in the most constructive way possible,

Then, the replacement of that negative feeling with a positive feeling of liking for your fellow man and pleasure with yourself for having achieved release without having hurt anyone else. This is a big step forward in your own emotional balance as well as in taking the strain off the heart.

The next step is to prevent the explosions that can occur through those small irritations that have accumulated during the day at work, fuelling any irritations that may develop on returning home.

Making a peace place

If you have problems both at home and at work, it is important not to let them build one upon the other thus making the sum of the whole greater than the sum of the parts. Identify a place between your home and your work and call it your 'peace place'. Choose a common, a park or a tree-lined road – a place that has an immediately pleasing effect on you. Leave your transport and stay there for at least ten minutes on your way to work and for the same period on your way home, or longer if your work day has been very fraught. All this will add at least another twenty minutes to your day, but years to your life expectancy. So it is well worth it.

Use it as a place where you reduce your anger and, before you leave, consciously renew your calmness and contentment. Walk off the frustrations and then let the calmness develop. This is now a well-tried technique and has saved patients from operations for gall bladder disease and other ailments that have been due entirely to the high build up of stressors overlaid upon stressors until the defence and immunity systems of the body have been unable to cope and illness has resulted.

Releasing anger at a half-way peace place is the ideal as you then arrive home having largely shed the frustrations, worries and irritations of the day. However, this may not be possible if you commute a long distance by public transport or if there is just no suitable place available. Patterns of anger release that have been tried out successfully in these circumstances are:

1 Going straight into the garden on arriving home and

104

digging or hoeing for half an hour before becoming involved in the worries of your partner or your children.
2   Taking the dogs or yourself out for a walk for half an
hour after arriving home.
3   Doing a routine exercise workout as your first priority.
   Families quickly accept these patterns as part of a person's unwinding process, and they have the added advantage that both partners, although in the home together,
have time to adjust to this change without compounding
each other's burdens at once. A cooling down period has
been provided for both. On the other hand, some people
find that they need to unload problems verbally and to yell,
rant and rave. This is wholly understandable. It is much
more of a continental pattern, but, if channelled, would do
no harm for those of us who really feel like exploding.

Rather than taking out your anger on humans you can use a   *The screaming*
bush or a tree. You can yell and rant and rave at it until you   *tree*
have exhausted and cleared your anger safely without any
danger to other people or yourself. It has been tried and
found effective. It also makes a good listener to your ideas
and arguments when you need to get something out and
there is no human companion ready and willing to listen.
There is something about a tree that is companionable and
that gives a sense of stability and peace. People tell me that
they have found it so.

With these sorts of releases actually working, the rapid   *Prevent anger*
reaction of the anger pattern will recede. This provides a
short time-lag in which to begin to apply preventative
techniques. One of the best is calming breathing (see page
109). It is easy to learn and simple to apply and it is very
good at dampening down the stress response. You can
literally breathe your way through difficulties and no one
will be any the wiser, other than to marvel at your new-
found self control. Once you have mastered this, you are
sufficiently cured to be able to use the time-honoured
formula of counting to ten before replying. That is a much
simpler method, but it will have little effect for you until
you have served your apprenticeship at anger release and
control. When you progress to this you are indeed handling
your stressors remarkably well. But now is the time to aim
at preventing them from starting in the first place.

Prevent your stressors from beginning

Delegate
Decide each day what you alone must do. Delegate the rest to others making them alone responsible for seeing that each task is done properly.

Master time
Put down everything you must do yourself in your diary – even the telephone calls – and allow plenty of time for them. Do not clutter the diary, and give youself time for the inevitable eventualities. This will cut down your perpetual rush.

Reward yourself
Give time to yourself once a week, even if after work. Visit a museum and sit and look at only one or two things. Go to a lunchtime concert. Let calmness steal over you just for a while.

Cope more easily with waiting
There is always something you wish you had had the time to read. Carry it with you, then you will (maybe in time) look forward to periods of waiting instead of resenting them as a waste of time.

Personalities with moderate stress risk
These are the strictly precise and the socially dependent.

Strictly precise We will deal with the strictly precise first. Your stress risk is only rated as moderate because the way in which you organise your life leaves very little to chance. You do not really like change and so you shun circumstances that might lead to it. You like a settled routine and so organise things in such a way that everyone fits in around it. You are fairly resistant to alcohol and may well be reasonably abstemious, so you do not have alcoholic problems to contend with.

What would be high stressors for you would be those unforeseen happenings which throw your well-organised life out of balance. These could be redundancy, a major illness, a break up in the family or a new boss who throws your routine out at work. These you would find very hard to take. It is difficult for you to relax, but the dampening down of the stressors is absolutely essential to save you from a stress illness if these disasters happen to you. Learn now the Relaxator Technique in the next chapter which is a combination of relaxing, autogenic training and visualisation. It will help to keep you stable through difficult periods.

You need affection and approval from people, and the mental stimulation of like minds. If you have a group of friends both at work and at home who are highly supportive, you will be able to tolerate quite high stressors, which is why your stress risk rating is only moderate and not high. The risk would only be high if for some reason you found yourself friendless and alone. You need people when you are troubled, and all your efforts should go into making and keeping deep friendships alive and working for you. To this should be added a wider circle of lighter relationships. Make a card index of all the people you know at home and at work, and those with whom you have had no correspondence for some time. Next buy a stock of postcards, which take even less time to write than letters, together with the necessary stamps. Now you are ready to pick up the threads of acquaintanceship and turn them into friendships. People like being remembered and they like hearing from you. Even if you get no reply at first, do not give up. Keep writing interesting little snippets of news and you will eventually get your replies. Develop a close circle of friends from among people you like and who live near enough to drop in. Invite them in for a drink, coffee or fruit after an evening meal, or for a quick one-dish meal at a Sunday lunchtime. It does not have to cost a lot, in fact it is better that it is cheap or others might feel that they cannot compete with the high standards you set. So keep it informal because you are developing friendships and that means giving your full attention to the people, not the food or the drink or the impression you are creating. If you are alone, you will be depressed, so move on next to Chapter 13, *Getting the Emotional Balance Right*, which deals with handling depression and then come back to Chapter 8 for your relaxation techniques.

The socially dependent

CHAPTER 8

Stress reduction techniques

This Chapter has two main parts to it. The first deals with First Aid techniques that are designed specifically to help you – if you are in Stage II Stress – to reduce your arousal and tension levels during the day, whether you are at work or at home. Your time is probably precious, so these First Aid techniques are headed two minutes or five minutes so that you can choose the one for which you have time available. They are all short-term answers to the problem of tension, but if they are practised frequently during the day, they become preventative techniques as well.

The second part deals with long-term curative techniques that will keep tension levels under control. You will then be able to switch off the stress response at will, leaving it always available at full power to be called upon when you need it in an emergency or crisis.

Breathing

You probably will not have noticed but we breathe in different ways according to what we need for what we are doing. When we are asleep, our breathing is deep, slow and rather forceful – you can always hear when people fall asleep. When we are under pressure, the breathing is shallow and fast and we use only the tops of the lungs. When we are really relaxed, the breathing is slow, rhythmic and very quiet. Anger, especially when being repressed, gives a rapid irregular pattern. Listen to the different rhythms of people around you, and you will see what I mean.

So the way we breathe alters our systems from rapid to relaxed, and from relaxed to sleep. In changing from rapid to relaxed, the 'at peace' state is engendered and the distress response is dampened down to 'off'. Blood pressure, cholesterol count, and all the biochemical changes that have taken place, return to normal.

108

By using our own physiological ways of breathing we can steady the system, stop panic from mounting, or deal with a very difficult situation in which our blood pressure is likely to rise and make us hot, tense and uptight. By using the breathing related to the system 'at peace', you can count on reducing the pressure and remaining cool and clear headed. It is a useful first aid measure to get you through all kinds of difficult situations. Also, if you get used to using it three or four times a day, you will reduce your blood pressure and lipid count (the fats, including cholesterol circulating in the blood stream) and this then becomes not only a first aid measure but a preventative one that will keep the blood pressure down permanently.

Steady the system

Breathing techniques

Calming breathing

Sit back comfortably in a chair. Drop your shoulders down naturally and feel them widen from the spine outwards to your arms. This is to allow full, wide lung expansion. At the same time pull gently up as if a string attached to the top of your head is pulling you up. This is to expand the lungs upwards. Look straight ahead as if looking at a point on the wall opposite you. Make that position feel comfortable – do not strain at it. Now your whole chest cavity will be able to expand naturally and allow your lungs to fill with air from the top to the bottom. So, to recap. Sit comfortably with a wide expanded chest cavity, dropped shoulders and an easy feeling. Now take five slow deep but gentle steadying breaths. Having done this, you are ready to start the calming breathing.

Breathe in easily and gently to a count of three and out just as easily and gently to the same count. Think of the three lobes of a lung and give a count to each one. Keep it all very relaxed and gently expand the chest outwards rather than trying for depth of breathing. Remember that this breathing should not be noticeable to others, the only external sign should be your calmness. It is not as deeply relaxing as when you are practising a more advanced form of deep relaxation. It is an opportunity for quietly dampening down the stress response by saying to your chemical and nervous system in effect, 'There is no need to come to my aid. I am coping with this easily and calmly.' So breathe away gently and slowly, 1–2–3 in and 1–2–3 out. As this is gentle, expansive breathing you can keep it up, for example, throughout a difficult interview. Once practised you can dispense with the preliminaries and breathe away gently and calmly whenever you need to, regardless of where you are.

When to use calming breathing

- When driving in heavy traffic your pulse rate can go up to 136 and even higher. Bring it, and your blood pressure, down with this calming breathing.
- On courses that are designed to stress you.
- When facing something that you know will put up your blood pressure such as facing a difficult interview, making a speech, dealing with awkward people, chairing a stormy meeting.
- Whenever you need a cool clear head, as when being interviewed or taking a test.
- When facing a hectic day, particularly when you feel harassed and need to reduce the stress arousal levels, use it frequently.
- Whenever you feel yourself getting uptight, bring down the tension with this calming breathing.

Diaphragmatic breathing

In order to benefit from this it is probably better to practise at home at first. Lie down on the floor with a small pillow under your head and another comfortably under your knees. Place your hands flat across your stomach with just the tips of the fingers touching. Now bell out your stomach as you breathe in, and press your fingers down with flattened stomach as you breathe out. As the stomach bells out, filling the lower lobes of the lungs with air, your fingers will separate and be drawn well apart. They come together again as you breathe out. Practise this belling out and deflating, moving the stomach muscles and the diaphragm as much as possible, but keeping the shoulders and the tops of the lungs as still as you can, thus allowing the diaphragm to do all the work. When you have practised this well you will be able to do it anywhere without attracting attention.

Rhythmic circular breathing for sleep

This method of breathing is useful for those people who find it difficult to switch the mind off the problems of the day. The mind becomes anchored to the rhythm instead of the problems and so the natural sleep centre is encouraged to take over. Make yourself comfortable in the position in which you want to sleep because at the end of this procedure you will be asleep. Close your eyes and settle down for sleep.

110

Now breathe deeply but gently in the same way as you would for diaphragmatic breathing.

Feel the breath filling up slowly from the diaphragm through the chest to your mouth, then, as you breathe out, imagine yourself blowing the breath out of your mouth, round in a circle back through an imaginary hole in your tummy to the diaphragm. Then start all over again, up from the diaphragm, out of the mouth, and round down to the diaphragm. Take the rhythm fairly slowly. Now you understand the principle, try it. Breathe in from the diaphragm slowly through the chest to the mouth, counting to four and blow it out back to the diaphragm in another count of four. Pick your most comfortable, fairly slow, rhythm. The most important part of this is the full involvement of the mind in the circular process of breathing. Keep a mental picture of the circle in your mind and follow it round at all times, making sure that the mind concentrates on and thinks only of this circular rhythm. Then, as there is nothing more interesting going on, you will fall asleep.

I use this method to get to sleep and rarely have to go beyond ten circles before I succeed. You will find that your eyes will automatically follow the circle from the mouth out and back to the diaphragm, and this is good, showing that the mind is involved. If you do wake during the night, know that you can get to sleep again quickly with this method.

There are times when you will need all the energy you can get without switching on the stress response. Here is how to do it.

Breathing for energy

Picture your lungs and what you need to do. You have three lobes on the right side and only two on the left. The top lobe of this left side is the same size as the top and middle lobes of the right side put together. You need to fill all of these lobes with their full amount of oxygen, in order to allow the exchange with fatigue products. Breathe in slowly allowing the stomach to bell out first filling the lower lobes with air. Then aim to fill the middle lobes (including, on the left, the lower part of the top lobe) and lastly fill the top lobes allowing the shoulders to expand and lift. Do all of this to a count of five (about five seconds), and then hold the breath allowing the full interchange of oxygen and fatigue products to be carried out. Hold for five seconds if you can. With practice this can be extended two or three times. (Pearl divers and sponge divers develop the ability to hold their breath for very much longer than this.)

Now let the breath go very gently, holding the top steady and letting the lower lobes empty first, followed by the middle, and lastly the top. Pause for a second or two and then repeat. As you breathe in, realise that you are taking in a full amount of oxygen for the energy you need, and as you breathe out slowly 'see' the fatigue products ebbing away with the exhaled carbon dioxide. Repeat this ten times and do it consciously whenever you need extra energy.

First Aid
resources

These are tension reducers for particular parts of the body. The parts that are liable to become most tense are the shoulders and the back of the neck. Whether you are at home ironing or making the beds (very tension-inducing if you would far rather be doing something more interesting), in the office typing, writing reports or standing at a machine doing a continuous and monotonous job, your neck and shoulders can be tensing up until they feel as hard and as stiff as a board. You can feel this hardness with your fingers. The problem is then intensified as the stiffness of the muscles can often restrict the free flow of blood between the head and the neck – there is only a very small opening – and the consequence can be tension headache or migraine. So we need to reduce this tension several times a day. It is easy to do and takes very little time.

Stand up, stretch high, and then let your arms flop to your side. Let them hang loosely with shoulders dropped and loose. Straighten the spine, tucking the bottom under, holding the stomach in, and raising the head in order to make a clear passage for the flow of blood to it. Do not tighten the shoulders.

Take five deep breaths, each in the following manner. Breathe in slowly and gently for a count of four, hold it for a similar count, and then breathe out slowly for a count of four, dropping the shoulders further each time. You will begin to feel the area of the back of the neck becoming warm as the blood begins to flow freely again.

Now circle your head gently letting it drop forward onto the chest, rolling it gently over the left shoulder, dropping it back behind you, over the right shoulder and dropping forward onto the chest again. Carry out four of these circles to the left, then repeat to the right, breathing easily and gently throughout the exercise. Finally, lift the head easily on the neck, take a long steadying breath, and then return to your work feeling considerably less tired.

112

This can be done sitting in a chair and is a very useful tension reducer before a meeting at which you want a particularly clear head, in the middle of a harassing day, or when you feel irritations are beginning to pile up. They must not be allowed to accumulate out of control. You know now that this is the way to put up your heart rate, your blood pressure and your cholesterol count up, so this is the point at which you must take action to dampen them down.

Head clearer (two minutes)

Flop back in your chair. Take a first deep breath in and now breathe out fully as if you were a balloon deflating completely. Go down with the deflating balloon. Allow your lungs to refill without any effort on your part. You are concerned with deflating yourself and driving out all the tension with the exhaled air. As you repeat this cycle you will feel yourself becoming more floppy with each deflating breath. As more of yourself goes limp and the irritation and tension leave you, you will find the head getting clearer and clearer. After two minutes take a deep energising breath, feel alerted, and breathe away quietly and normally. Now go to your meeting with a clear head and a refreshed mind, happily unhampered by tension.

Do this during a break during the day such as a tea break. You will not have realised that your shoulders are tense until you stop and attempt to loosen them. You can in fact do this sitting down but it is better to stand to give free movement to your arms.

Shoulder release (three minutes)

Stand. First stretch high with both arms and then with each separately. Now stand with feet just a little apart to give you a good firm base and raise your arms in front of you to shoulder level. Then loosely and lazily swing them down and behind you and then back again. Do not put any effort into this as you are loosening shoulder joints and reducing tension. Effort only increases tension. So slowly and easily let them flop down and back, forward and up, repeating these swings rhythmically ten times. Finish by moving the shoulder joints in a vertical circle, five times forward and five times backwards for each shoulder, and they will be much less tense and much easier to live with.

This technique is the important rag doll-like flop that switches off the stress response completely. You will recall that the stress response alerts the Sympathetic Nervous System which is the activating system that makes every-

Rag doll (five minutes)

113

thing else in the body go faster. This technique calls up the opposite system, the Para-sympathetic, often called the 'rest and digest' system. As the two cannot operate together at the same time, the stress response, sensing the resting state of the body, realises that there is no emergency and switches itself off. So, this is a very useful stress reducer at lunch time or at the end of a day before facing the journey home.

Sit on an armless chair. Do ten deep, slow diaphragmatic breaths and with every outgoing breath breathe out quite forcefully, deflating like a balloon, and begin to flop forward at the head and neck. Gradually flop further forward with each breath out letting the shoulders and arms fall further and further forward until you are hanging limply from the waist like a rag doll. Hang there for a minute or two and then come up very, very slowly. Rest your head back on the chair and breathe slowly, gently and easily with your hands resting limply and lightly on your lap. Sit quite still like this for a s long as you can manage, though four minutes is quite long enough to reduce the pulse, heart and blood pressure rates. When you are ready to take up the threads of work again, take that deep energising breath, and you will feel alert and freed from tension.

The Relaxator Technique
This technique is a combination of relaxation, autogenic training and visualisation (these techniques have been developed by Western physiologists as being suitable to a Western way of life) and the three have been incorporated into one system by the Stress Foundation. Research into the many different methods recommended for stress control suggests that it is rare for one particular technique to provide all the answers. We are all different with differing needs, and evidence suggests that the best method will usually be a combination of techniques that have a proven history of effectiveness. Those that the Foundation has chosen to combine have just such a well tried record.

The progressive relaxation method developed by Edmund Jacobson, an American Professor of Physiology.

The autogenic training method developed by

114

Johannes Schultz, a Berlin Neurologist.

Visualisation which is the picturing in the mind of
a peaceful and calming place.

Visualisation has been used for centuries and its origins are really lost in antiquity. The progressive relaxation and autogenic training methods have been developed particularly for those of us who live in the West. This is not in anyway to decry the long established and respected methods of the East. Every civilisation develops its own techniques suitable for its own people and their cultural beliefs. Once learned, the programme takes only fifteen minutes and is best carried out every evening after the day's work. We will do the relaxation part of the three way programme first.

Muscles are powered from the motor control area of the brain and, in addition, each group of muscles is powered from its own motor area. Even if you only think about doing something, this thought is translated into activity and your muscles react. So, if you are constantly thinking of what you have to do, your muscles are tensed up ready to do it. Power is permanently switched on and you are, as it were, burning up your electricity and running yourself at a loss. The control for each muscle as it is actually moved is in its own fibres. You are only aware of sensation when a muscle is moved and not when it is relaxed and so you have to learn how to recognise the signals that muscles are switched on too high, when they do not need to be.

Progressive relaxation

When we are asleep, the power should be switched off in all muscles. We need power only in those groups of muscles that we are actually using, so by switching off the power in other groups that are not needed you can save vital energy, prevent fatigue, and reduce wear and tear on yourself. This is how it can be done and worked into a busy schedule.

Learning differential control

First learn how to recognise how much effort you put into quite small movements. You do not need to make all this effort. You would be more efficient with only half the effort. Lie on a folded blanket or rug on the floor. Put a small pillow under your head and another under your knees to make yourself as comfortable as possible. Use the calming breathing to settle yourself, and then the breathing for relaxation which is breathing in slowly and gently and then expiring quickly, deflating fully and almost pushing the breath out of you. This is necessary because every muscle group will be tensed, even though you will not be aware of it, so consciously deflate yourself as in the breathing for the rag doll.

Switch off your right leg

Be conscious of your toes. Wiggle them slightly. Try to feel where their power comes from. Bend the foot slightly up feeling the source of the pull. Do you feel it only in the foot? Do you feel it in the leg? Even in the knee? Do the same now bending the foot slightly down. Remember that you are not trying to exercise, nor to relax. You are really on a voyage of discovery about yourself, trying to find out the source of power for each group of muscles in order that you can lessen the movement when full power is not needed. Move each muscle group in your toes, legs and up to your thighs several times, learning about them. Learn what moves them, where the movement comes from, and what they feel like when moved, and what they feel like when absolutely still. Then from the toes, become aware that the muscle groups are at rest. Become aware of the other muscle groups at rest as you trace them up to your right hip. Work only with this leg to start with. Do not consciously try to relax the muscles – just become aware that they are at rest and let it happen.

Autogenic training

Now breathe away gently and quietly as you are going to do autogenic training on that same leg. Do not, for the time being, think about any other part of the body. You are gradually going to become aware that your right leg is becoming heavy as limbs do when they are thoroughly relaxed. In order to let it happen, say to yourself, 'My right leg is becoming heavy.' Repeat this slowly to yourself 10 times over the period of a minute. This induces the switching off of that part of the motor area in the brain that controls the legs. It now realises that movement is not needed at present. If it is not getting heavy yet, repeat it for another minute or two. Then when it is feeling heavier than your left leg, say to yourself, 'My right leg is getting very warm,' in exactly the same way for the same length of time. Then do the same with the left leg. Now both legs should be feeling heavy and warm and pleasantly relaxed. Lie there remembering the feeling of really relaxed legs and do not attempt to do any more than this at first. We are not seeking full relaxation yet – just the knowledge and experi-

116

ence that we can switch off groups of muscles when we no longer need them for active use and at the same time produce an effect that feels good and pleasant. You can imagine how marvellous it will feel when you have progressed to the whole of yourself. It really is a thoroughly enjoyable, beautiful, rejuvenating feeling. So far, you have only spent about ten minutes, and for the next five minutes you now carry out the visualisation technique.

Visualisation

This technique varies from the very simple practice of mentally picturing your favourite peaceful scene to projecting pictures onto a screen. The latter might include, for example, pictures of cancer cells being attacked and engulfed by your anti-bodies in the blood stream. This is actually what happens and it has been established that actually 'seeing' it happening strengthens the actual happening, although it is not yet understood why. It is probably similar to the way in which, when we think about writing a letter, our arm and hand muscles start to 'fire' (which we can actually hear through a biofeedback machine) to prepare for writing. But let us deal here with simple visualisation to switch off the stress response.

Visualise a peaceful picture

You are lying quietly with heavy warm legs and breathing gently, easily and evenly. Quieten the breathing down now even further and allow your mind to linger on a scene that you find tranquil and peaceful. For me, this scene has elements of water and trees, and the colours are a mixture of quiet greens and blues. It is sunny, but not glaringly so, and the shadows of the overhanging trees are reflected in the water, and move gently as the water laps the shore. It is an idyllic place. Take a little time to think about yours. It should be a place that has significance for you. For me, water and trees have been important from my childhood. Water and trees. What are the important elements for you? Identify them, put them together and keep them constantly before you to feed your spirit during visualisation.

Getting up

After a session of relaxator, do not immediately leap up, but take up your activities again very slowly and calmly. If you do not need to rush around and work afterwards, do not take an energising breath, but stay at this slower tempo for the evening. You will find sleeping at night easier because you have switched off from the problems of the day. Do not take them up again until tomorrow.

117

The full
programme

The next night follow exactly the same routine but this time start with your arms and then include the legs. Start with your right hand if you are right-handed, or the left if you are a left-hander. When one hand is heavy, extend this to the whole arm saying, 'My right arm is getting heavy,' exactly as you did for your legs. Then move to your other hand and arm, and finally your legs. You end with visualisation. As you proceed you will find that the rest of the body automatically becomes heavy and warm without you actively thinking about it. After the arms and legs, you can turn your attention to the trunk. Start with the buttocks and follow exactly the same pattern as with the legs. Move one set of muscles on one side only, gently finding out where the controls come from. Are they in the buttocks only or do they extend to the back? Carry on exploring, moving the tops of the thighs. When you move these are the legs involved as well? Move both the front and the back muscles of the trunk. Do this with the other side, then both together, squeezing first the muscles in the buttocks alone, then in the front and then in the tops of the thighs. Then, after gentle breathing and feeling them relaxed, follow on as before with the autogenic training, feeling the whole area to be heavy, then warm. Let this heaviness and warmth now extend to the legs, and finally to the arms, ending it by visualising your peaceful retreat.

The following night it is the turn of the back. Settle yourself down as before breathing gently, easily and quietly. Begin very gently to move the different muscles in the back, up from buttocks to shoulders, feeling each set in turn, but making only very small movements. Then try to discover the muscles in the sides in between the ribs and at the base of the shoulders. Think how many different movements your back has to make and therefore how many different sets of muscles there must be. There are actually well over 1000 muscles in the body, and we tend to hold far too many of them taut and over-strung even though we actually need only a few. For example, do you actually need your shoulder and jaw muscles to write a letter? Follow this discovery again with gentle breathing and feel all those muscle groups relax. Then follow with autogenic training feeling them first heavy from the shoulders to the base of the spine, then warm. You will find by now that the heaviness and warmth are automatically spreading to the hips, buttocks and legs, and very likely to the arms as well. All this results from the brain picking up

118

signals that it is time to switch off. Finish with a picture of the peaceful you, in your own peaceful place.

We treat the stomach separately from the trunk as there are so many muscles involved and discovering them is important. The stomach suffers particularly badly in the state of stress, and learning to relax and calm it can make the difference between suffering and escaping an ulcer. Lie very comfortably, knees slightly flexed over your small pillow and breathe gently and quietly. Now begin to move the stomach muscles gently, starting at the lowest level and finishing at the ribs, afterwards trying one side and then the other. Move the muscles inside as well. The stomach and the intestines are muscular and you can learn to relax all of them and thus prevent the 'knots' of fear and panic and the gripes of anxiety. Having discovered all the different small movements you can make, slowly reduce them and relax them, and follow with autogenic training, feeling the whole area becoming heavy, relaxed and then warm. *Stomach relaxation*

You may well need to give the whole available time to the stomach, especially if you suffer from gastritis, dyspepsia or ulceration. Keep the entire area relaxed and pleasantly warm and think to yourself, 'My stomach and all my insides are relaxed and working smoothly. I feel pleasantly warm all through.' Think it through several times, savouring the feeling. Let that feeling extend to the back and the whole trunk area. Finish with visualisation as before.

We have left the head and neck till last because it is very difficult to relax all the scalp, face and neck muscles when one is concentrating on the rest of the body. Now it is their turn. Lie comfortably with a small cushion under the nape of the neck so that head and back are in a straight line. Bend the head slightly back feeling the pull in the back of the neck. Is the back involved at all? Involve the back gently, and then only the neck. Move it forward and identify the control. Move it to the left and right and feel the controls. Now relax it and feel all the muscles relax right round the neck, sides, back and front. Realise how many unnecessary muscle groups you usually involve in your everyday movements. Remember to keep the intensity of these movements down and use only the smallest amount of power. Now feel them all relaxed and then follow with autogenic training and finally visualisation. *The head and neck*

119

The face

This should be part of everyone's beauty treatment as it relaxes the frowning and worry lines which give the appearance of ageing. Wrinkle up the forehead. Where are the muscles that you are using? Now frown. Can you frown without using any other muscle power? Close the eyelids fairly tightly. Are you using neck muscles? Look up and from side to side using the eye muscles. Are your jaw muscles being used as well? Now use your eye muscles differently. Look into the distance, follow a bird swiftly across the sky, look at a pin point, watch a slow ball bouncing from side to side, and look back into the distance again. Now relax all those muscles.

Next close your jaws firmly, and then let them fall open again. Do this several times, learning which muscles you use and where they are. Do you need to use them all for talking at length? Think about it. Now smile in different ways involving different muscles. Pout, and then relax all the muscles of the face and the eyes. Relax them and feel them heavy and warm. At this stage we are left with the muscles of the scalp. Try to move each ear separately. Try to move the skin at the back of the head from the top of the neck over the top of the head. Relax them all, thinking of all the muscles involved in the neck, face, eyes and scalp. Feel them all pleasantly relaxed, first heavy and then warm, and finally, finish with visualisation.

The forehead: keep it cool

Behind the brow are the frontal lobes of the brain, the site of the will and the intent to act. It pays to keep that cool, unless you are doing this just before going to sleep.

Now you have gone through the whole of the body, taking one night for the right leg, one for the left, one for each arm, finally progressing to the head and neck on the eighth day. After this you will find that you are able to do both legs together, and then both arms, and by the end of the second week you can relax, and make any part of yourself heavy and warm at will.

CHAPTER 9

Driving yourself to drink and other drugs

If you have come straight here from the end of Chapter 2 you are worried that you are already in Stage III Stress. You are probably feeling very down, exhausted, and afraid that you will never again be energetic and on top of the world, coping with everything that you once did so easily. But you will. You also do not know how on earth you got into this state. Often when we have been coping with everything so well, some minor thing will happen that proves to be the straw that breaks the camel's back, and we go to pieces. It has happened to me, and it happens to most people who lead hectic lives, although you would never know it. Let me give you some examples.

The first case was Sarah, a 42-year-old wife and mother with four children. Her husband was a bricklayer, at times unemployed in the winter. She worked as an office cleaner for twenty years, working at night and taking on an extra morning shift when her husband was unemployed. She had boundless energy, was always cheerful, ran her home and the family like clockwork and was unworried by problems – 'Not more than usual in life, I suppose'. Then she slipped on a patch of polish and broke her arm. It was slow to heal and prevented her from working. She became very depressed, down and tearful. Her family, sympathetic during the broken arm period, gradually lost patience as the weeks became months, telling her to stop feeling sorry for herself and to snap out of it. Her doctor told her that if she went back to work she would soon regain her former good spirits. This she did, dragging herself through the days and feeling suicidal. She had no energy to do anything, and just felt that life was not worth living. That is all past history and she is now fine, and her usual cheery self.

Sarah's story

121

Gregory's story	The second is Gregory. He was 'head hunted' from the EEC to head up an ailing industry. The salary offered was inviting and he brought his family back from Brussels and entered the cut and thrust and insecurity of industry in this country. After a year of struggle he gradually became more and more morose and felt that he just could not cope. Commuting was a nightmare, the unions were proving difficult and he felt alienated from his immediate senior staff. He felt a failure. Now he is thriving and attacking life at his previous pace and demonstrating the technical grasp and know-how for which he was originally chosen.
Anne's story	The third is Anne. She was a very bright 28-year-old in public relations, married to a lawyer with a good practice and lifestyle. She left him for a rising young star in advertising, an affair that lasted only four months. So she threw herself into work and – living in a bed-sitter – socialising, leaving herself little time to think of the ruined marriage, the short-lived affair and the depressing bed-sit life. She looked terrific and impressed everyone by her vitality, energy and the sheer amount of work she got through. She was promoted, but then she was left to manage the firm herself during the holiday period and that was when she suddenly panicked. She could not think, could not remember, and the thought of having to see a client gave her uncontrollable fits of shaking. She feared that she was finished and would only be able to do a shop assistant's job to bring in the rent. But she is now a partner in the firm and no one will ever know how near she was to complete breakdown.
Time to stop	Sarah, Gregory and Anne had all been living and working for years at the very top of their stress energy levels. Sarah – 'I must keep going day and night for the sake of the family.' Gregory – 'I have to make a success of this having uprooted the family from their home and friends in Brussels.' Anne – 'I mustn't allow myself time to think about the mess that I have made of my life. Press on faster and faster.' If you are in this sort of state, the first thing to realise is that, like Sarah, Gregory and Anne, you have been taking far more out of your fuel tanks than you have been putting back, and they are now empty. Hence the panic attacks, the loss of energy, and the feeling of despair, as all your faculties stop. Now you have to stop and let the body refuel, and the brain rest, and the whole recover. You

122

need a 'pit-stop' for repair and maintenance, which means that you, like any other engine, have to be taken off the track for a while.

First of all, you really do have to stop completely. If you *The pit-stop* have two, or preferably three, weeks leave due to you, take it immediately. If not, you will have to manipulate some sick leave. The minimum must be two weeks, and having arranged that, this is what you do.

Tell your family that you are preventing a heart attack (which is probably true) and put yourself on absolute rest. This means total bed rest. Lie propped up comfortably with plenty of pillows and for the first day or two do absolutely nothing but sleep. Do not look at the television, do not listen to the news and do not read. If you like, have some gentle soothing background music, but the whole idea is to give the body and brain – which includes the senses, sight, hearing and speech – nothing whatsoever to do except rest. So sleep or rest comfortably with your eyes closed. Do not have visitors and do not have the family fussing round you. All you need is plenty of fresh fruit juice beside you, a light diet (just a little of whatever you would like), but no spirits or alcohol of any kind, and nothing heavy like steak and kidney pie or suet puddings. Stick to eggs, fruit, cheese and salad accompanied by wholemeal bread and butter.

On the third and fourth days, if you are beginning to feel *Do not even* rested, take to a little light reading. The purpose is only to *think* let the mind and body rest and daydream in another world, and so it must not be anything you have to think about. Light, frothy books or humorous tales are ideal. At the end of the week, try a little light television for a short while, but do not watch anything that you have to think about, and certainly nothing to raise your temperature. In the second week, get up in the afternoons and take a little gentle exercise like a short stroll in the garden, or round the block if it is not too far, but there must be absolutely no work and you must go back to bed after tea. By the end of two weeks you should be feeling increasingly rested and more confident that you will be able to cope at full strength again by the end of a month. If you do have to go back to work at the end of the two weeks, do the minimum at work and then come back to your rest in the evenings. At the end of the first week back at work, use the weekend break to get as much fresh air as possible, and for gentle walking. In the second week back, in the evenings, read and practice the First Aid and relaxing techniques set out in Chapter 7. At the end of the month you should be feeling that you are gaining control again.

Vitamins

Now a word about vitamins which you must start to take immediately and keep taking for at least this first month. You will need Vitamin B Complex. Make sure that it is B Complex which will include vitamin B12 as well as the more usual B vitamins. These have been put out into the system with the stress chemicals and used up during the state of continuing stress. You must replenish your stores of these. You will probably only be able to get these at health food stores. At the same time get some vitamin C, the anti-infective vitamin. The body does not store this vitamin and uses it up rapidly when in stress, so you will need high doses. Get the one-gramme, effervescent tablets and take one every day. They can be fruit flavoured and are pleasant to take.

All work and no play

Now, although you are feeling much better, you will still have some way to go to restore yourself to full health. You will need to restore your emotional and social health, making sure that work takes up only a part of your time. In each 24 hours you probably spend eight in bed, which leaves you with 16 hours a day. Now do the quiz on page 39 *Taking stock and stopping Stage II Stress*, and see where your life is out of balance, and then make out an overall plan for your 16 hours. Remember yourself too. You will need time to refresh and to re-create yourself emotionally. It is so easy when you feel better and you find the energy beginning to build up again, to become once more the workaholic that you probably were before your system went on strike and cried 'enough'. Think of yourself as a very precious piece of machinery which you would never run into the ground. So, how are you going to 'drive' yourself from now on?

How do you drive yourself?

What do you drive? A Rolls? A Ford Escort? A souped-up Mini? What you drive very often determines how you drive. A souped-up Mini is usually seen going flat out, weaving in and out of the traffic; a Rolls, on the other hand, is never driven flat out and there are always reserves of power and energy which, at the touch of the accelerator,

124

will produce a turn of speed that will leave all others standing. Why is a Rolls never driven flat out? Various reasons offered me recently include, 'You don't need to, there's plenty of acceleration to get you out of trouble if need be;' 'It's a piece of high-precision engineering and built to last;' 'It's very expensive, only a fool would burn that engine out.'

Think about those statements – 'There's plenty of acceleration to get you out of trouble if need be'; 'It's a piece of high-precision engineering and built to last'; 'It's very expensive, only a fool would burn that engine out'. Now, think how you drive yourself? The human system is a valuable piece of high-precision engineering; it must last a lifetime for there are no second-hand models, and it would be foolish to burn it out. And you do not have to drive yourself flat out, because there is plenty of accelerator to get you out of trouble. At a touch of your accelerator – the human stress response – large reserves of power and energy are immediately at your disposal. You would be wise to drive yourself as if you were driving a Rolls – with a light toe.

Plenty of acceleration in hand

As we have seen in Chapter 2, the human stress response has an effect on us that is many ways similar to the effect of the accelerator on the engine of our car. It is by no means an all-or-nothing response, but produces energy in direct relation to the amount of pressure that is exerted upon it. If faced with the rush hour we might think, 'Rush hour – challenge – it's going to be murder today.' We are, as it were, pushing the accelerator right down to the floor. The stress response will leap into action to get us out of the crisis. But we really do not need the resulting surge of power and energy just to sit in the car and wait. All that energy will be misdirected into frustration, tension and anxiety. Situations like the rush hour, which we cannot alter, need the reverse of an accelerator: they need the acceptance of things as they are. We need to apply our energies to the problem of making the situation work for us. For example, time is usually very important for us and if we have an hour's journey, that hour is precious. Could you balance an early night with an hour's earlier start, miss the rush hour and do an hour's work in peace before the rest of the staff arrive? Many firms are able to stagger hours, so work out the hours that would suit you best

Stress is our accelerator

125

without the hassle of the worst of the rush hour and ask if that is acceptable to your organisation. If, on the other hand, you are a housewife and mother, do you need to keep the accelerator hard down on the floor all day? You could stagger your work hours as well.

The rhythm of running and rest

Think of yourself as a powerful and expensive Rolls or Bentley. You have a powerful machine in your hands with plenty of reserves to call upon if you need to. You only have to learn how to drive it, how to control it and how to maintain it; how and when to let it cool down if you have done the unforgivable and driven it too hard; where to fill it up and with what (any old fuel will not do, see Chapter 12 on food) and you have to know when to rest it. The rhythm of running and rest is important, isn't it? Running keeps everything tuned up, but running continuously wears an engine out.

You are a Rolls

By now you will have understood the implications but may be thinking, 'I am not a Rolls – more like a souped-up Mini.' You are a Rolls; in fact, you are much more powerful. We have over 50 per cent more of everything than we need. We have more brain cells than we will ever use; two kidneys, and we need only a part of one to function well; two lungs, and again we can function well on a part of one; we can dispense with part of the intestine and stomach; the heart functions in spite of considerable damage, and you only have to see the liver of an aged alcoholic to see that very little of it can have been functioning for years. We have far greater reserves and resources than we can use in a lifetime, but we must learn how to control the energy supplies. Stress management should really be called energy management. You have seen yourself what happens to energy in Stage III Stress – it is non-existent, isn't it? When we have rested and recovered our stocks again, we can afford to drive with a light toe knowing that, at a touch of the accelerator, we have surges of power available to get us out of trouble. Our options are very clear: drive flat out all the time, use up all the petrol in the tank, burn out the clutch and possibly end up by crashing head on into a wall, or drive as a Rolls should be driven, well under control and in quiet confidence that it is capable of meeting any demands that may be put upon it. The Rolls is too valuable to do otherwise – and so are you. Think of yourself and how very nearly you burned yourself out.

126

Preventing Stage III Stress from occurring again, therefore, involves driving oneself intelligently and paying attention to the system and its needs. By paying attention to the system and understanding its needs, we can prevent a great deal of illness. For example, when we have the accelerator flat down on the floor to get us out of trouble in an emergency, no attention is paid to anything else. All other functions stop, and everything else is sacrificed to the paramount need to get quickly out of danger. Would you want to eat while driving in a race at Brands Hatch? Hunger, thirst, the desire for sex and the operation of all other bodily functions stop while we are driving flat out, in order to allow the body and mind to concentrate without distraction upon the challenges we are facing. But, supposing you are not really in danger; you are not racing, not dangling on a rope on the north face of the Eiger, nor making a tricky parachute descent? In fact, although you are driving yourself flat out, you are not at all in a life or death situation. You have got your accelerator flat on the floor – for what? A normal day at the office or at home? Calm it down, take your foot off the accelerator and return all the bodily functions to normal. Remember particularly that when you are flat out the normal working of your digestive system will have been suspended, so if you are going to have a meal it will not be digested properly and you will have dyspepsia, gastritis or gastric ulcers. No wonder you feel so awful.

Drink and drugs

Many of us I know, when trying to deal with a highly stressed system and lack of response, think that we need a stimulus, and so we have a drink, and then another and another as the memory of what was troubling us begins to fade. Alcohol is, after all, an anaesthetic – and a good one. So we need to know how far we can benefit from it without becoming an alcoholic.

The short answer to this is, yes it will. Alcohol is a sedative and an anaesthetic just like chloroform, ether, morphine or marijuana. It relieves our worries, anxieties and fatigue because it anaesthetises the brain, starting with the frontal lobes just behind the forehead. This is where our seat of awareness is located. So if we are aware of anxiety and fatigue, and after one drink feel a little less anxious, we go

Will a drink help?

127

on to another and another. These put the frontal lobes out of action, and we are soon no longer aware of anything except what we see and what we are doing and feeling at the moment. If we are just having a few drinks with friends, we probably feel terrific. The only snag is that if we need a fully alert brain for work, we have not got one even though we feel marvellous and are quite sure that we are efficiency itself.

Does it do any harm?

There is no evidence that light social drinking has any injurious effect on the body, and so you will find many people who will say that it does not do you any harm. In fact there is a book written by a doctor entitled *Drinking is good for you*. He obviously knows little about the brain. The danger of alcohol is that, like many other drugs, it is habit forming to particular personalities. Unfortunately, we cannot say for certain in advance who is going to get 'hooked' on it.

Light social drinking

The definition of 'light social drinking' fits those of us, probably the majority, who drink because it is the custom among our friends, or to relax after a heavy day. The term 'social drinker' fits any one of us who drinks moderately, who has no tendency to increase the level of drinking, who can 'take it or leave it' and who could give it up.

Heavy drinking is dangerous

Heavy drinkers are not alcoholics. They may drink heavily because their friends and their lifestyle set a fast pace. They could moderate their drinking or cut it out completely if need be. In other words, they remain in control. It is, however, dangerous because heavy drinking leads to health problems and to mistakes and accidents at work and on the roads.

The compulsion to drink to oblivion

Alcoholics tend to increase their drinking over time. First of all they find that they cannot stop at just one or two drinks, then they develop the compulsion to drink and they may either drink consistently or alternate between steady drinking and short periods of abstinence after which they start again and cannot stop. They are the 'uncontrolled, compulsive drinkers'. Soon, drink dominates their lives and they are quite unable to stop by themselves. At this stage it has become an illness, and the sufferers need help, not recriminations. We have about 600,000 alcoholics and about one fifth of these are women.

128

It can be fatal because it anaesthetises the brain and lowers our awareness of danger. *Alcohol is a dangerous drug*

1 in 4 pedestrians killed are 'over the limit'.

1 in 3 drivers killed are 'over the limit'.

It is dangerous because of its effects upon the brain, and as the amount of alcohol drunk per head in a country goes up, so the rate of entry to mental hospitals for alcohol misuse goes up. The figures below show the increase per head in pints of alcohol taken by individuals over the age of 15, and come from the Brewers' Society. The figures for hospital admissions are from the Department of Health and Social Security.

Year	Consumption per capita aged over 15 years			Admissions to mental hospitals for "alcohol misuse"
	Beer	Spirits	Wine	
1960	192.5	3.9	4.7	2,479
1970	228.3	4.7	8.1	8,708
1980	267.7	11.2	19.2	17,358

As the rate of drinking goes up, so also does the death rate from cirrhosis of the liver (and its hardening due to alcoholism which prevents it from functioning normally). *Resulting deaths*

This death rate went up from 56 to 69 per thousand between 1960 and 1980 alone. Between 1970 and 1980 the increase was approaching 60 per cent.

So alcohol can kill us and can send us crazy. Is there anything else? Well, yes, there is quite a lot more. It has produced convictions for drunken driving that have more than doubled in the period we are looking at and which stood at 122,259 in 1980. It is closely associated with crimes of violence, terrorism and hooliganism, and no one knows the figures for these. Those who are married to people with serious drinking problems know only too well the rapid change that can take place and turn a normally sunny, caring person into a dangerous and violent aggressor. This is what happens if alcohol has deadened the frontal lobes of the brain, which should be keeping the personality intact. *It can make us violent*

One drink is fine, two are alright. If you do not have to work, a glass of wine with food is civilised, and a party is *So to sum up* great fun if it can be held at the weekend and there is time to recover before Monday morning. More than this during the day affects your brain and your performance. Those who cannot function without a drink are in serious trouble, because they are hooked on a killing drug. It is like everything else in the body, isn't it? A little does nothing but good, like stress itself. Too much can kill you.

Do you have a drink problem? First of all take note of how much you are drinking, and its effects on you. Here are the conditions to expect:

Merry	2–3ozs whisky or 4 × 12oz bottles beer
Clumsy	5–6ozs whisky or 8 × 12oz bottles beer
Dizzy	10ozs whisky or 4 quarts beer
In a stupor	1 pint whisky or 6 quarts beer
Dead drunk	1 1/2 pints whisky or 9 quarts beer
Dead	Over 1 quart whisky

You do have a problem if:
- You cannot wait till 6pm for that stiff drink to get you unwound.
- You have to have a drink before you make that important telephone call, see that difficult client, or carry out any of the duties associated with your job.
- You habitually drink by yourself.
- You have to have a drink in the morning to get going.

For those with a problem, it is vital to stop drinking. After a period of abstinence the physical symptoms of perhaps upset stomach, sore throat and changes in your liver function, which you may not be aware of, will clear up and the nervous symptoms of irritability, failing memory and loss of concentration will then gradually get better. You will need the active help and support of family friends and colleagues in your effort. Your GP can often be a tower of strength, giving you injections of vitamins to help your overall health. Furthermore, if the withdrawal symptoms are bad he can help with medication, and if the psychological effects of withdrawal are too much for you to cope with, he will be able to recommend a therapist who will help you over this early stage. Identify a soft drink that will suit you; if you are a gin-and-tonic drinker, try exactly the

130

same drink without the gin. If a Scotch drinker, try dry ginger ale. They look the same to other people and to you – only you (and the barman) know that the spirits are missing.

Keep up a good mixed diet with plenty of vegetables for your mineral shortages (see Chapter 12) and take a course of vitamins, particularly vitamin B Complex for your nerves. With good food, vitamins, reassurance and help from your family and friends, you should be able to stop drinking without going into hospital and without drug treatment. When you would have your drink beside you, have that soft drink you decided upon, and for drinking with meals, join the new tycoons and have a Perrier water.

After a period of abstinence you will feel better, but drinking is probably the way in which you attempted to cope with the demands being made upon you. You will find these lessened as the effects of alcohol on the brain wear off. You will be more clear-headed and able to think things out better. You will not make so many mistakes, so work will be more interesting and rewarding. Nevertheless, when demands pile up, you will be tempted to drink again and blot them out. So learn the techniques in Chapter 7 and prevent the tensions from building up. By keeping the arousal levels down to manageable limits you will no longer be tempted to blot them out because you will have tranquillised them the natural way.

And how do you cope with stress now?

Learn the relaxation technique outlined in Chapter 7 and use it every morning and night to calm your system down while you are weaning yourself away from dependence on alcohol. Then use it every evening to relax thoroughly and return the over-active system to normal. Read, *How do you drive yourself?* earlier in this chapter. Drive yourself like a Rolls Royce, knowing that you are back in control of the very cream of engines – man. We have the most intricate, the most complex and the most creative self-regulating machinery ever devised. It really is worth looking after.

Drinking safely depends on several factors. I would include the following safety measures:

Drink safely and enjoy it

1 *Line the stomach before drinking.*
Alcohol is taken straight into the bloodstream from the lining of the stomach. So line it with anything that

will coat it. Milk is good, olive oil is marvellous if you can take it, but a well buttered slice of wholemeal bread will suffice.

2 *Drink slowly*

Keep to one in each hour and do not join in fast rounds of drinks. Immediately alcohol is taken into the system it is, like anything else we take in, broken down chemically. It is first oxidised and changed into carbon dioxide and water, and the carbon dioxide is excreted by the lungs. So drink very slowly to allow this breakdown to go on.

3 *Eat at the same time*

Keeping the stomach lined will slow down the absorption of alcohol.

4 *Dilute alcohol well*

Drink your favourite drink well diluted with fruit juices, water or other mixers. Keep the concentration down for the sake of your brain.

5 Know what is your safe daily ration.

6 Never have one for the road. Allow at least an hour before driving.

What is safe?

The rates are different for males and females because women, and we do not yet know why, get cirrhosis of the liver much more quickly than men and become alcoholics at an earlier age on exactly the same amount of alcohol per body weight.

The safe daily rate for men is: as given in *That's the limit* published by the Health Education Council.

2 pints beer OR

5 measures spirits OR

5 wine glasses of wine OR

5 glasses of sherry

With this amount, you will be 'under the limit' and safe to drive if you are an 11 stone man. If you weigh less than this, keep to under 2 pints or 4 of the others, and drink slowly.

The safe daily rate for women is:

1 pint beer OR

132

2 measures spirits OR

2 wine glasses of wine OR
glasses of sherry

Safe, that is, to prevent cirrhosis of the liver. However, as the above rates will deaden the frontal lobes, it is probably wiser not to start at lunchtime or more stress will be induced in the afternoon. Actually, it is better not to start at all. If you can meet your demands through the natural means outlined in Chapter 7, and drink pure fruit juices, you will be healthier, more clear-headed and less stressed.

You may be taking other drugs at the same time that you are drinking. It would be much better if you did not. The group of drugs usually prescribed for stress, that is those used to control anxiety and to induce sleep in the over-anxious, are Benzodiazepines. They act as depressants on the central nervous system by blocking off the stimulation from our arousal system. Exactly how they do this is still unknown. As we can control this arousal ourselves by the techniques outlined in Chapter 7, particularly by the calming breathing when we feel our anxiety mounting, we should not have to take drugs for this. *Other drugs*

It is important for every one of us who is stressed and leads a pressured life, to know as much as possible about the drugs that might be prescribed when help is needed. We will then be more able to make up our minds whether we should take advantage of them, for how long and how to come off them quickly and safely.

The most common Benzodiazepines are given below, first their real clinical name, and then their trade name in brackets.

(Chemical)	(Trade Names)
Chlordiazepoxide	Librium
Chlorazepate	Tranxene
Clobazan	Frisium
Diazepan	Valium
Flurazepam	Dalmane
Lormetazepam	Noctamid
Nitrazepan	Mogadon
	Serenid-D Serenid
Oxazepan	Forte Serax

Temazepam	Euhypnos Normison
	Cerepax Levanzol

Some of these are given for daytime sedation and some are given as hypnotics to induce sleep at night. Many people believe that this group is not habit forming, and that there are no withdrawal symptoms, so they can be prescribed with safety. This is, unfortunately, not true. Tolerance can occur, which means that the nervous system gets used to the drug and will need more of it to be effective in relieving the state of anxiety. Withdrawal symptoms can also occur, which means that when the drug is stopped, the body, having become used to functioning with it, cannot function efficiently without it. Symptoms are likely to be anxiety (for which it was prescribed in the first place), restlessness, and less commonly, a feeling of nausea and difficulty in sleeping. There may also be tremors and occasionally delirium.

These drugs are useful in the treatment of mental illness to damp down high excitability and hypomania. They should not be prescribed for our general emotional problems though doctors are often faced with a dilemma. They want to be as helpful as possible to their patients, and their patients have come to expect that a pill will make them better, and so expect a prescription. But there is rarely a need to prescribe for daytime sedation, except during a period of high grief after the loss of a spouse, for example. Then it should only be used for two weeks, just to tide the patient over the very worst period of loss. But even then, social support is more effective, longer lasting and has no ill effects.

Drugs for sleep These drugs are often prescribed as hypnotics, that is, to help people to sleep at night. Again, the advisability of this is now being questioned. The reasons are that the people for whom they are prescribed are often in middle age or older, and go to their GP complaining of having 'fitful' sleep at night. Research on sleep patterns, which is now extensive, shows that people in their middle years and later do not sleep deeply all night. There are many periods of light sleep when they often waken. This is not 'fitful' sleep as many describe it, it is good sound sleep with a few waking periods of short duration followed by further sound sleep. So perhaps these facts should be more readily avail-

134

able to GPs who may not be up-to-date with the latest research (and no one could possibly be – there is so much of it) and information and reassurance given to patients instead of drugs which they will never be able to give up as their 'fitful' sleep pattern will return as soon as they are not drugged. In later middle age, the waking periods are longer, but the sleep is wholly adequate.

So if Benzodiazepines are used for periods of high distress they should only be taken for very short periods of one or two weeks at the most. If you have been on them for longer and want to come off, talk it over with your doctor and get his help. He will be only too happy to help you do this and this is how you do it. First of all learn the relaxator technique thoroughly and practise it to calm down the anxiety state or depression from which you are suffering. Next learn the rhythmic breathing to induce sleep and practise this while you are still on your drugs. Then tell your doctor that you have mastered these techiques and are ready to come off the drugs.

Drugs for one or two weeks only

If you have been on them for longer than a month you will need to come off them gradually. The dose should be reduced by half a milligramme only and stay at this level for a week. Then reduce by a further half milligramme for the following week, and so on until you have cut out the dosage completely. In this way there is no rapid withdrawal, the system becomes used to smaller and smaller doses, and you will be building up your skills in handling your stressed system by natural means. Give yourself a special treat every Sunday morning as you reduce the dose for the coming week and you will then get positive pleasure from the reduction. You can do it and you will feel so delighted with yourself.

Come off gradually

So turn to Chapter 7 now and learn the techniques, then reduce the dose and get that marvellous system of yours back to normal.

CHAPTER 10

Developing a balanced lifestyle

This is the chapter on lifestyle and tells you how to develop a balanced, whole way of life which will let you get the best out of yourself, and also delight your family, friends and acquaintances. We are all destined to be so much more dynamic and effective than most of us are, and happier and more at peace with the world. But we cannot be when feeling low, depressed, anxious, fatigued or only half alive. So the following chapters deal with just these problems in more detail. They deal with fatigue and tell you how to build up energy and stamina through the right kind of exercise and food. Chapters 13 and 14 deal with the problems of depression and anxiety and how to handle them in order to return your emotional balance to an even keel. The last Chapter of this section, Chapter 15, tells you how to get the social balance right, which cannot happen unless you are happy and content within yourself. So it is, in fact, all about you – giving yourself the time and space to be yourself. You have so much more to give to others when you are happy and content within yourself.

So far we have recovered from Stage III Stress and in the process have realised that we can cope with the stress in our lives better and more effectively through an informed understanding of the problems facing us, and through relaxation techniques rather than through alcohol and other drugs. In addition, we have been reducing our blood pressure and our lipid count (which is mainly affected by stress) and we can sleep at nights. We are now driving ourselves in a more relaxed way and in consequence are able to make full use of our accelerator, our stress response, in real emergencies. We also know that to stop Stage II Stress, we have to pay attention to developing a balanced way of life; and that is exactly what this chapter is all about – developing a lifestyle that will give us health and vigour till the end of our days. We humans do not have to develop arthritis and rheumatism – we do not have to develop cancer and other ills – and we certainly do not have to become senile. We can retain full health and vigour, remain energetic and live to well over a hundred, if we know how to go about it. The key is to keep in mind how we are built, and the purposes for which we were built. If we were to use a race horse as a plough puller, or a shire horse for racing, we could expect trouble from them, if not heart attacks. Horses are built for different ways of life, and so are we. It is worth taking a little time to think out the sort of lives we were built for.

To a surprising extent man still has much of the bodily constitution, the physiological reflexes and the emotional drives that we inherited from our Palaeolithic ancestors. We should not be surprised at this as there are only 100,000 generations between the earliest man and you and I. That is not a lot when we realise that fossil records of life go back six hundred million years to the Palaeozoic Era and we developed only half a million years ago. So we are the new boys on this earth, but the most adaptable species yet. We can and do adapt to many different environments: tropical forests, arctic snows, high mountains, plains and deserts. But we do not so much adapt to, as interact with an environment, making alterations to it to suit ourselves.

Our traditional lifestyle

But some environments we have influenced do not suit us. Perhaps the most alien environment of all for man, other than that of space, is Western industrial society. Here he lives in a centrally heated, electrically controlled box; he is transported in small motorised boxes to other centrally heated, electrically controlled boxes for eight hours of work; he is then transported back again to sit for hours every evening in front of another electrically control-led box, not even moving for food which is brought to him on a tray. I find it hard to believe that this is really true, but this is what the social surveys tell us. If it is true for you, then alter your lifestyle without delay for it will be doing you no good at all.

Man is an explorer with an in-built curiosity to satisfy. Traditionally, we are movers. We are built to run, to leap, to lope (not jog) with a long easy stride for miles without tiring; to walk, to fish and to hunt: in short, to move. To make sure that we do what we are built to do, we have an in-built curiosity that drives us to explore our environment.

We are explorers and movers

137

Every mother who has had the contents of her cupboards spread all over the room can testify to this. We have inbuilt storage systems of energy to provide the fuel for all this movement and an accelerator (our stress response) for a shot of extra power and energy to meet exceptional demands or to escape from danger. Interestingly, the more energetic we are, the stronger we become in muscle power, in arterial circulation and in heart stroke. Energy begets energy. The more we partake of physical activity, the more energy we develop. The more we use our brain power, the greater its development. Conversely, the less we use any part of our body, the less we are able to do so. For example, some people believe that sexual activity ceases with the menopause, and they stop. When they discover that sexual powers are still strong in the centenarians who have never stopped, they find it difficult to start again. There are people who have made their first parachute jump at 60, and learned to ski at 65. There are people who have taken up riding, gliding and similarly active sports after they have retired and have had the time to devote to them. They have kept themselves fit and active, which is just what we are going to do. The answer is constant and regular use. Use ourselves as we are meant to be used, and we can live with health and vigour and energy as long as we have a mind to. However, read Chapter 11 before starting.

You can live to be 100

How long could we live if we were really fit and vigorous? If our hearts were strong and our arteries unfurred and all our organs in good shape, would we have to die at the traditional three score years and ten? Metchnikoff, a Russian writer, after studying the lives of many centenarians, was so struck by their mental and physical vigour that he became convinced that man was meant to live very much longer than he usually does. He seems to have been proved right by the many people who are now remaining vigorous and fit, some well into their second century. The earliest documented case that I know of is Thomas Parr. He entered into the history books because Charles I sent for him to find out how to live long and well. That was in 1635 when Thomas was 152 years old and as fit as a fiddle. Unfortunately, after wining and dining only too well at Court that night, he died – of a surfeit of unaccustomed rich food and drink. So be warned, do not over stress the system when you get to 152. Incidentally, his post-mortem showed that he could have gone on for many years. Unfortunately,

Charles I did not live very long after that either. Another Charles, Charles Thierry, did though. His biography shows quite clearly that his doctor attributed his long life to his habit of going for very long walks every day no matter what the weather. When he was 103 he developed influenza. This left him depressed as influenza always does, and he found it difficult to recover his lost energy and was inclined to sit about and brood. His doctor prescribed a resumption of his daily walking, and he very quickly recovered his former vigour and vitality.

How many Centenarians?

There are well over 12,000 people in their second century in the United States. This is to be expected of this very health conscious nation, but we are catching up. Ten years ago we had only some 200 centenarians and today there are over 2,000 who are now being studied by the Royal College of Physicians. How much do we already know about this? We know that it is apparently healthier to live in the south of the British Isles, and that it helps to have had a good education, presumably to be able to read the health information. It also helps to have a family history of longevity. Activity and exercise appear to be all-important as we have already emphasised. We also know that women have nine times the expectation of living to over 100 than men. This is supposed to be due partly to their higher pattern of activity in the home, as well as having a genetic advantage over their menfolk. In a recent, large American study of energetic centenarians, the one common factor that emerged from every case was that they did not worry about the things that they could not alter.

How you do it

The American Centre for Consumer Health Education has developed the following questionnaire to obtain a 'Life Score'.
    It takes in all the known factors:
        Family history
        Exposure to infection
        The stress of change
        Weight and diet
        Exercise
        Attitude to medical care
This assessment is only suitable for adults with no chronic disease and who are not suffering from heart attacks or strokes.

139

Lifestyle assessment

Conditioning exercise

Count the total number of minutes in a week in which you take conditioning exercise, ie brisk walking, hard tennis, squash, jogging or any exercise that raises the heart beat (pulse) to 120 beats per minute (not bowling, golf or ambling).

If your minutes per week total:

Less than 15	Score 0
15–29	+2
30–44	+6
45–74	+12
75–119	+16
120–179	+20
180 or more	+24

Weight

Check your weight against the tables opposite. Heights are without shoes and weights are in pounds.

(For women between 18 and 25, subtract one pound for each year under 25) If you are overweight by:

0–5 pounds	Score 0
6–15	−2
16–25	−6
26–35	−10
36–45	−12
46 or more	−15

Diet

If you eat a balanced diet – one that includes vegetables, fruit, bread and cereals, protein foods and dairy products, score +4. If you stay away from saturated fats and cholesterol mostly found in animal fats, score +2.

Smoking

If you do not smoke at all, score 0. If you smoke only a pipe, score −4. One cigar is equivalent to one cigarette. If the number of cigarettes you smoke each day is:

1–9	Score −13
10–19	−15
20–29	−17
30–39	−20
40–49	−24
50 or more	−28

If you smoke at all and take birth control pills, score −7.

Men 25 and over			
Height	Weight for frame		
Feet Inches	Small	Medium	Large
5 1	112–120	118–129	126–141
5 2	115–123	121–133	129–144
5 3	118–126	124–136	132–148
5 4	121–129	127–139	135–152
5 5	124–133	130–143	138–156
5 6	128–137	134–137	142–161
5 7	132–141	138–152	147–166
5 8	136–145	142–156	151–170
5 9	140–150	146–160	155–174
5 10	144–154	150–165	159–179
5 11	148–158	154–170	164–184
6 0	152–162	158–175	168–189
6 1	156–167	162–180	173–194
6 2	160–171	167–185	178–199
6 3	164–175	172–190	184–204

Women 25 and over			
Height	Weight for frame		
Feet Inches	Small	Medium	Large
4 8	92–98	96–107	104–119
4 9	94–101	98–110	106–122
4 10	96–104	101–113	109–125
4 11	99–107	114–116	112–128
5 0	102–110	107–119	115–131
5 1	105–113	110–122	118–134
5 2	108–116	113–126	121–138
5 3	111–119	116–130	125–142
5 4	114–123	120–135	129–146
5 5	118–127	124–139	133–150
5 6	122–131	128–143	137–154
5 7	126–135	132–147	141–158
5 8	130–140	136–151	145–163
5 9	134–144	140–155	149–168
5 10	138–148	144–159	153–173

Work out the amount of alcoholic beverages you drink *Alcohol*
each day. One drink equals one and a half fluid ounces of
spirits or eight ounces of beer or six ounces of wine. If your
drinks are larger, multiply accordingly. If your average
daily intake of mixed drinks, beers or glasses of wine,
totals:

141

0	Score 0
1–2	+1
3–4	−4
5–6	−12
7–9	−20
10 or more	−30

Car accidents

The car is the number one cause of accidental death, and seat belts can save about 50 per cent of car accident victims. Most people think they wear seat belts more than they actually do. Take a minute to work out, honestly, how often you wear yours.

If the time you wear a seat belt is:

Less than 25%	Score 0
About 25%	+2
About 50%	+4
About 75%	+6
About 100%	+8

Stress level

One way of measuring your stress level is to look at the changes in your life. Add your points for the life changes on page 52 in Chapter 3.

If your score is:

Less than 150	Score 0
150–250	−4
250–300	−7
More than 300	−10

Personal history

If you have been in close contact for a year or more with someone with tuberculosis, score −4.

If you have had radiation (X-ray) treatment for tonsils, adenoids, acne or ringworm of the scalp, score −6.

If you work regularly with asbestos and do not smoke, score −2.

If you work regularly with asbestos and do smoke, score −10.

If you work regularly with vinyl chloride, score −4.

If you live or work in a big city, score −6.

If sexual activity has been frequent and with many different partners (for potential of venereal disease), score −6.

For women only (risk of uterine cancer): if you began regular sexual activity before the age of 18, score −1.

For each parent, brother or sister who had a heart attack before the age of 40, score −4. *Family history*

For each grandparent, uncle or aunt, who had a heart attack before the age of 40, score −1.

For each parent, brother or sister, with high blood pressure requiring treatment, score −2.

For each grandparent, uncle or aunt, with high blood pressure requiring treatment, score −1.

For each parent, brother or sister, who got diabetes before the age of 15, score −6.

For each grandparent, uncle or aunt who got diabetes before the age of 25, score −2.

For each parent, brother or sister, who got diabetes after the age of 25, score −2.

For each grandparent, uncle or aunt, who got diabetes after the age of 25, score −1.

If you have a parent, brother or sister, grandparent, uncle or aunt with Glaucoma, score −2.

If you have a parent, grandparent, brother, sister, uncle or aunt with gout, score −1.

For women: if your mother or sister has had cancer of the breast, score −4.

If you have had the following check-ups, score the points *Medical care* indicated:

Blood pressure check every year, score +4.

For women only (risk of breast cancer): self examination of breasts monthly plus examination by doctor every year or two, score +2.

For women only (risk of cancer of the uterus): cervical smear every year or two, score +2.

Tuberculosis skin test every 5–10 years, score +2.

Add and subtract all the points you have scored. *Your life score*

Total points scored	. . . . .
Now add	+200
Your life score	. . . . .

A life score of 200 is average. If you scored above 215, you have an excellent chance of enjoying better than average health. A score of 230 or more means that the odds of a healthy, long life are overwhelmingly in your favour. A score below 185 means that your probability of a healthy life is decreased, below 170 you should consider that you are heading for serious illness.

How long do you have? Another way of showing how decisions affect your health is to make a rough estimate of your life expectancy. The table below translates your life score to estimated life expectancy.

Your health	Life score	Estimated life expectancy	
		Men	Women
Excellent	230+	81+	86+
Good	211–229	74–80	79–85
Average	191–210	67–73	72–78
Below average	171–190	60–66	65–71
Poor	170 or less	Less than 60	Less than 65

You may be worried that you have relatives who have died young with heart attacks, or that there is diabetes in the family. Do not worry about this, for all it means is that if you let yourself get into Stage III Stress, the part of the body that takes the strain is likely to be the same as the rest of your family. But you are not going to let yourself get into that state, are you?

Your lifestyle to prevent diabetes

You have groups of cells in the pancreas that manufacture insulin which breaks down the sugar in the system into a form of glucose which the body can use for energy. It is possible to overload these cells and strain them. We get all the sugar we need from natural foods, fruit and vegetables, and we have no need to take it in in the form of the sugar in the sugar bowl which does absolutely nothing for us except to overload our insulin-producing cells, So, if you do have a family history of diabetes, cut out all the sugar in your diet as far as you possibly can. Try to drink mainly pure fruit juices without added sugar. It is difficult to avoid sugar in our food today as all manufacturers add it to everything from baby foods to soups. So read the labels carefully when you are shopping.

Keep your weight down to the average for your build and height which is explained in chapter 11 and 12, and do not worry. Stress is often the trigger for the development of diabetes, so read carefully *Taking stock and stopping Stage II Stress* on page 39 and make sure that you develop a balanced lifestyle. This means giving yourself emotional satisfaction as well as physical exercise and ensuring that you have good friends in which to confide. If you have let yourself get into Stage II Stress, then follow the directions for coping with this in Chapter 9. There really is no reason to develop illnesses just because they are part of your family history. Decide now that you will remain fit and well.

You may well have a relative who has had a heart attack, and perhaps even one who has died from one. It does not mean that you will too. All it does mean is that you are forewarned that strain in you may well be felt in the heart and circulation instead of in some other part of the system. Your need is to strengthen the heart and the circulation system so that it is wholly equal to any strains that you may put upon it. Being forewarned, you will also keep those strains down to a manageable level.

Lifestyle to prevent a heart attack

The underlying cause of the majority of coronaries (coronary thromboses) and strokes (cerebral thromboses) is that the arteries, instead of being fit and toned up with smooth clean walls, are flabby and furred up like household water pipes in a hard water area. Then fats (fatty acids, oils and glycerols including cholesterol) that are circulating in the blood stream, stick to these receptive walls and interfere with the circulation. If we hardly ever do anything more than shake a duvet or ring for a secretary, the circulation is slowed down and a small clot (a thrombosis) may form and lodge at a narrow junction in the heart or the brain causing a coronary in the former or a stroke in the latter case.

So keep that circulation moving.

1 Reduce your anger and irritation. These increase your blood pressure. See Chapter 7.
2 Keep those arteries smooth and cut down their furring with toning up exercises. See Chapter 11.
3 Keep that circulation moving. Walk.
4 Reduce your heart rate and blood pressure during the day with first aid tension reducers. See Chapter 8.
5 Enjoy lean meat instead of fat.
6 Get used to vegetable oils (like sunflower) for cooking instead of lard.
7 Keep to a normal weight. See the chart on page 141. Being either too thin or too fat puts an unnecessary

strain on the system. In the first case you have no reserves to fall back on when you become ill, and in the second you are giving the lungs and heart too much to carry.

8 If you must smoke, enjoy a pipe, leaving it unlit for periods and do not inhale the smoke. Cigarettes will not do you much good.

9 Do not jog, unless you are very fit. Loping, a gentle long stride, is better than jogging the system about, especially if you have to run on hard surfaces.

10 Try out lots of vegetable dishes, and try out the nutty flavour of 100 per cent wholemeal bread made from stone-ground flour.

11 Walk, walk, walk.

Start to walk briskly every day

If you were to say that you could not alter the whole of your lifestyle in one go and ask what you should make a start on, my answer would be without a doubt – walk. Walk briskly everywhere, every time you have the chance. This is not just for the sake of your circulation and for toning up the arteries which as we have already seen is crucial. It is also to burn up those fats that have been called up by the stress response and are already circulating in the system. So another crucial point is to keep your worries and anxieties down to a manageable level. All the research on the different treatments of anxiety and depression shows that of two groups, one of which had psychotherapy and the other daily exercise, the movers did better and stayed better. It is important to note that the movement was 'conditioning' movement: brisk walking, swimming, etc. Even strolling gently in the open air in pleasant countryside at least reduces worry. So do build this into your lifestyle. If you can only manage 15 minutes a day, build in an hour or two's brisk walking at the weekend.

Why worry?

One of the main factors that characterises the lifestyle of the vigorous centenarians is that they can shed unprofitable worry. They all have this ability in common. Many say, 'Well, there is no point in worrying if you can't change it, is there?' In other words, they use worry in the positive way in which it is meant to be used – that of motivating one to solve the problems. If the problem is one that cannot be solved, they give it up, and turn their minds to something more constructive. Would we could all do this. We live in an anxious and anxiety-making age and many of us have let

146

our natural resilience go. The next two chapters will help this because activity, as we shall see, reduces anxiety, and the foods that we eat will increase our resistance. But more than that, we have to tackle the anxiety and the depression we feel now, before we can stress proof the system properly. This we will tackle in chapters 13 and 14.

So after all our research into what makes for a healthy and vigorous life, are we any nearer making a plan for a vigorous lifestyle? Yes, I think we are. To do this, we have to put together what we know of how we are built to function physiologically and biochemically. We have to know what the hazards to a vigorous long life are, such as the cancers, the infections, heart diseases and psychosomatic illnesses. More importantly, perhaps, we have to keep in mind our defence and immunity systems to all of these illnesses. You see, we are marvellously designed. If you knew of all the defence mechanisms in the body, you would wonder how we ever become ill. You would marvel at the way we break down every drug that enters the system, including alcohol and tobacco smoke; the way we waft out infection from the lungs; our amazing fighting cells, which are doing battle every day undetected by us; and the lymphatic system that drains away all the dross of the battles. More extraordinary still is our system of recognition of friends and enemies. This is the reason not all of us develop cancer and similar illnesses. 'Foreign' cells are recognised and engulfed and this is most obviously demonstrated when modern medicine tries to foist on to us a different piece of skin or heart or lung from someone else. The main difficulty is not the six-hour long operation: it is to get the body to accept what it immediately recognises as foreign.

A plan for a lifetime of vigour

So, in our lifestyles, it seems to me that the most important factors are:

1 To develop a lifestyle which most closely follows the pattern for which we are built.
2 To develop a lifestyle which enhances and makes even more effective our defence and immunity systems.

For, let us face it, we cannot avoid contact with infection, nor should we wish to do so as this is how we develop our antibodies against it. Most of us enjoy a party and like a

147

drink. All we have to do is to give the body time to break that drink down before we have the next one. Some of us, in fact four out of every ten adults, enjoy a cigarette or a pipe and cannot give it up no matter how hard they try. Do not stress yourself about this.

Take the stress out of smoking

Look at smoking sensibly. Some people become very distressed at not being able to give it up, but smoking is not the only causative factor in cancer or heart disease. There are very many others. So think sensibly about how you live and where you live. Smoking is, I suppose, one's own internal air pollution. Now, if you live in a smoke-filled town, beside a motorway or close to a power station you would be crazy to add to an already overloaded (not in your favour) health hazard. On the other hand, if you live in the country, or at the top of a hill, then you will suffer less pollution from a cigarette than your non-smoking friends living in a big city will from their environment. So look around you and take a sensible view. If, after reflection, you feel it is better to cut down, then this is how to do it:

1 Find out the tar and nicotine content of your favourite brand of cigarette and compare it with the others. Change to the lowest tar and nicotine content you can find. Research shows that after changing, smokers do not smoke more, they often smoke less.
2 Do not smoke right to the end of the cigarette. Most of the drugs are in the butt. Smoke only two thirds of each cigarette.
3 Reduce inhaling. It is the *smoke which enters your lungs* which does the damage. Blow it all out – better still do not take it in.
4 Postpone your cigarette. Buy your packs later and later. Keep them locked in a drawer, not at your elbow. Promise yourself a cigarette after the next meal. People often find it easier to postpone than to cut out completely. Remember that one cigarette increases the heart rate from 72 to 88 and over. Blood pressure increases and the fats in the blood increase in concentration. So it does not help heart disease.
5 Why not try a pipe? It is something to do with your hands and mouth. It can remain unlit without you looking silly and it is certainly less toxic than cigarettes.
6 Remember that most doctors have given up smoking. If you want to know why, go to the nearest hospital and ask to see specimens of lungs with carcinoma of the bronchus. It may be just the motivation you need to help you stop.

148

Why not have another shot at giving it up?

1 Plan when you are going to do it.

2 Plan what you are going to do with the money you save and where you are going to keep it.

3 Write down when you smoke – after food or when you pick up the telephone. Plan what you are going to do instead – perhaps chew a licquorice stick or chew gum. Have it ready. Clear the house of ashtrays and cigarettes and all reminders of smoking. Prepare your friends and colleagues well in advance of the stopping date so that they do not encourage you to smoke.

4 Make the stopping date a very special day for you. Try the weekend and plan an outing somewhere special. It is better to be in different surroundings on the first day.

The plan for energy

1 Take half a glass of hot water with a dessert spoon of lemon juice in it on waking. This clears fluid and toxins from the tissues and tones up the system.

2 Eat breakfast every morning. This releases energy gradually throughout the morning.

3 Walk briskly for fifteen minutes to the station or bus or from a car park to work. This activity speeds up the system naturally and keeps the circulation distributing energy to the brain and all the organs long after you have stopped.

4 Eat a light lunch with fresh vegetables, salad or fruit and anything else of your choice. There is something in fresh vegetables that we do not yet understand. Freshly harvested green vegetables fed to guinea pigs kept them free from tuberculosis; and other freshly grown foods protect us from specific infections although we do not yet know the reason why. So we will play it safe and have freshly grown foods whenever possible.

5 Drink only fruit juice or water at lunchtime if you have to do brain work in the afternoon.

6 Do something every week which you enjoy. Give yourself a small treat. It may be naughty, like a cigar after dinner, a whole bar of milk chocolate, or reading an interesting book instead of doing the ironing. Plan this in your diary and, when achieved, plan the next thing to look forward to with pleasurable anticipation. We all need to be able to look forward to something good.

7 Do not worry about the things which cannot be altered. If you find your worries going round and round, carry out the calming breathing and stop them. Do this every time you feel unconstructive worry building up.

8 Give yourself at least a quiet half hour. This is your own peaceful time when you put your feet up. Do not let anything or anybody disturb it. Let the mind wander where it will and daydream.

9 Go out for a ten-minute walk before going to bed. This movement will help you to sleep.

10 Practise the relaxator technique before going to bed in order to sleep easily.

If we analyse this plan, we see that we have energy and vigour from the release of minerals, vitamins, amino acids and carbohydrates for the morning with the topping up of these for the afternoon to keep up the energy levels for the day. We have a clear brain for problem solving in the afternoon and evening. We will have good circulation from the brisk walk to ensure that all the vitamins, minerals, etc reach every part of the body including the brain. The heart is being gradually strengthened through the 'conditioning element' in the walk because a pulse rate raised to 120 or over during brisk exercise develops the heart into a stronger condition. Rest, in peace and quiet, even for half an hour, balances the brisk activity and restores calm to the system, and the emotional satisfaction of doing something that you really enjoy and have looked forward to is an essential balance for our hectic lifestyle today.

In trying to understand how we function and to meet this as far as possible by our own lifestyle, we are after something much more important than just helping ourselves to adapt to the environment that we have made, however lethal it is. We are giving everyone the knowledge to enable them to live as fully and as creatively as possible and to fulfil their own potential. We were all destined to be so much greater, so much healthier and so much happier than most of us are today. We all have enormous potential if we can only tune into it, and the following chapters are designed to do just that. First, let us rebuild and restore our physical balance.

CHAPTER 11

Getting the physical balance right: exercise

We are built to move, and until about forty years ago everyone did. Children walked to school and people walked or cycled to work. Housewives walked to the shops. It seems odd to realise it now, but a distance of a mile, taking just twenty minutes to walk, was thought of as 'just down the road'. Why have we changed so much in so short a time?

Now children ride to school, workers are transported to work, shops have come under one roof and have installed trolleys and lifts, and there is little need for us to use our legs and no need at all for the majority of the population to really use their backs or muscles. The consequence is that if we dig the garden, attempt to move the furniture, carry a sack of dog meal or even bend to tie up a shoelace, we can slip a disc. And 'weekend athletes' have coronaries while 'keeping fit'. How unfit can we allow ourselves to get? It is small wonder that we are fatigued most of the time after what our forefathers would think of as a moderate day's work. We will soon not have the strength to sit at our desks without backache. Indeed, this is already the case for some. We are literally driving ourselves to failing joints and coronaries. Most people over the age of 21 now living in the industrial West with its own particular lifestyle, have arteries which are 'relaxed' instead of being shiny, toned-up, elasticated and smooth. Globules of fat become easily attached to their linings and this condition (called Atheroma) is reversible until about 26 years of age, after which the sedentary pattern of life creates the conditions for our 'way of life diseases' with heart attacks leading the field. But we are not going to succumb to these because we are going to start to move and get ourselves fit again. We are going to discover that surge of energy and feeling of

Driving to a coronary

151

well-being which comes from being really healthy and having an enlivened circulation coursing through our veins and arteries, pumped by a strong and virile heart.

We should have the strength, the endurance, speed and agility to play several hard sets of tennis, to swim several lengths of a pool, or to walk for 20 to 30 miles a day without tiring. This is what we are built for – long, sustained free movement. That we do not do it is at the root of many of the ills today such as heart disease or arthritis.

What can we expect to achieve from starting activity?

1 It will lessen our chances of getting the 'sedentary' diseases as we get older – arthritis, rheumatism, slipped discs, hypertension, heart disease and strokes, diabetes and depression. All these occur less frequently in the really physically fit.

2 It will give us energy. The entire circulation is rejuvenated; it courses along carrying oxygen to every part of the body. Oxygen cannot be stored and the difficulty in a sedentary life is to get sufficient oxygen to all the body tissues where food is burned up. Food and oxygen together make for energy.

3 It will give us strength. The heart muscle is strengthened and becomes more efficient. Its own circulation improves and we can accomplish tasks with less fatigue.

4 It will give us flexibility. The strength and flexibility of our joints, our tendons and ligaments are improved and this makes it unlikely that we will slip discs or damage our joints while gardening, carrying or moving things.

5 It will lessen our fatigue. The efficiency of the lungs increases. This means that more oxygen is available to the tissues and there is a greater and more efficient exchange with carbon dioxide and fatigue products.

6 It lessens the risk of heart disease. The fats in the circulation are lowered, reducing the risk of Atheroma and coronaries.

7 It will trim the figure. Exercise stimulates the rate at which the body works (our metabolism). This speeds the burning up of sugars and fats in a natural way and keeps the body trim and looking youthful.

8 It stress proofs the system. It reduces stress by burning up the biochemicals, fats and sugars released by the stress process, and counteracts depression and so lifts the spirits.

9 It allows relaxation to occur naturally and so induces rest and deep sleep at night.

10 Last, but not least, it rejuvenates us and leads to a

152

feeling of euphoria, or the 'high' of well-being. This is why once you start you will feel so fit and full of energy that you will want to continue.

Real fitness for the type of life we want to lead really goes beyond what we normally think of as 'fitness' in the physical sense of the word. For our kind of lifestyle we need the energy and the stamina to keep up an intellectual staying power for the whole of our working lives. We need to continue to develop our social relationships, to take part in sporting activities with friends, and we need sufficient additional energy to enjoy life with our families. In other words, we need a fully balanced life and this takes full health, energy and vigour.

What is fitness?

Many of us after a long day of commuting and high mental pressure feel tired at the end of the day. We feel strongly that we need rest, not activity. But remember that for most of us our bodies have been at rest all the night before, and for most of the day. It is only our brains that have been active. They should now be given an opportunity for rest, and our bodies should now become active to restore the balance. The tiredness we feel is caused by an unbalanced system. There will be the biochemicals of the stress process which are there ready for physical action and which only physical activity can rapidly and efficiently disperse. We have become so brain-washed into believing that the antidote to stress is relaxation, that the physiology of the stress reaction is forgotten. The object of the acceleration of body and brain is activity; not just for speed, but for power and additional strength as well. In other words, the biochemical and nervous system changes that take place are the preparation for both physical and mental effort, but primarily for physical effort. If only one aspect – the mental – is used, it creates an imbalance in the system that can only be put right by physical activity. Relaxation should then follow this physical activity when it will occur naturally and completely.

Energy is created by breaking down the chemicals in the food we take in daily in the form of carbohydrates, proteins and fats. These are broken down in the presence of oxygen. The chemicals not immediately needed for energy are stored for future use. Oxygen, although essential for the use and conversion for storage of chemicals, cannot itself be stored. It must be taken in continuously. We do this by

Why do we feel tired?

153

breathing, but if we are just passive breathers using only the tops of the lungs (as we do if we are sitting all day), the oxygen does not reach all parts of the body where food is burned. Oxygen, together with food, combines chemically to form energy. The problem lies in ensuring that sufficient oxygen reaches every cell in the body for total energy release. When we achieve this, our fatigue vanishes.

Activity produces energy

Most people produce sufficient energy for their daily activities of walking, talking and thinking. It is when activity becomes much more demanding, such as having to run for a train or a bus, that we realise how unfit and how lacking in energy we really are. We are really fit when we are able to maintain prolonged work without undue fatigue. Exercise improves the circulation, increases the oxygen carrying capacity of the blood and the number of capillaries, and increases cardiac efficiency and output. The heart becomes stronger and develops a wider, slower stroke, increasing the circulation with little effort.

Am I only passively fit?

There is passive fitness described above, where no effort is being made to keep the heart, lungs and cardiovascular systems in good working order. Only the daily routine demands of a sedentary job are being made upon the system. The body then deteriorates, arteries fur up, the circulation slows down, and even the bones lose their strength and begin gently to decalcify. This deterioration will continue unless some effort is made to improve the respiratory and cardiovascular systems.

Or am I muscularly fit?

Due to the importance given to body building by Charles Atlas in the 1930s, the isometric or isotonic system of muscle development gained popularity. One can have muscular tone and strength without having strengthened the heart, lungs and circulation. Isometrics is the strengthening of muscles by counter pressure, eg you can sit in a chair and press the buttocks down while at the same time placing the hands under the seat and pulling upwards hard. These exercises should not be used in place of a programme of positive fitness.

Positive fitness is stress proofing

This is, as the name implies, more than an exercise prog-

154

ramme. It is proofing the entire organism against stress, thereby making it easier to handle adversity – emotionally, intellectually, physically, socially and spiritually. In other words, it is aimed at achieving a healthy mind in a healthy body. Results are not going to come quickly – in fact, it is essential that you proceed slowly and build up energy and strength gradually.

There should be a number of safeguards built in to any exercise programme that protects the passively fit from injury when they first start, because it is easy to injure muscles and a heart that has done little more than tick over for years past. Many join a keep-fit class and start skipping and running and doing hard floor exercises, and end up with sprained ankles, pulled muscles and sometimes even a slipped disc. *Play safe*

So, think about these warnings:

1 Do not start by jogging or running – get the heart fit first.
2 It is better to start your exercise programme at home and not at a club where you might attempt to compete with others before you are fit enough.
3 Build up towards hard exercise sessions gradually.
4 Start every session by warming up as you see the athletes do. This gets the circulation into the muscles. Cold muscles are easily damaged.
5 Keep to a schedule to monitor your gradual fitness and do not be tempted to hurry it along. You have been a long time running down; take your time over building up.
6 Once started, keep it up. Fifteen (preferably 20) minutes a day is better than two hours once a week. One hour twice a week is also better than two hours once a week.
7 Cool down after every session. Watch the athletes on TV. At the end of a race, they do not stop at the tape, they slow down gradually to a walk and keep moving as the body cools down.

First of all, have you any of the following conditions? *Check lung and heart conditions*
   – Asthma, or any chest complaint.
   – Diabetes. You will need more sugar if your activity goes up, so have your insulin/sugar balance checked.
   – A heart condition.
   – Aged over 40, and have done little more for years than drive a car, take gentle strolls and shake a duvet.

If you have, then the first thing you should do is go to your family doctor, tell him exactly what you intend to do, and ask him if your blood pressure and heart are sound enough to allow you to start. If you are cleared to start, it is a good rule to allow one month of conditioning for each year that you have been out of condition, ie have not been taking daily exercise at a brisk pace.

To find this out you have to know how fast your heart has to work to allow you to do more than you have customarily been demanding of it. This you can tell by taking your heart rate, felt as your pulse. To take your pulse:

1 Turn one hand over, palm facing up.
2 Line up the thumb with its first (index) finger, letting it lie on top of it in a straight line.
3 Place the index and middle fingers of the other hand on the thumb and follow its line back to your wrist.
4 There you will find your pulse, on the outer side of the wrist at the base of the thumb.
5 Press down gently and you will feel the pulse beating.
6 Now, using a watch with a second hand, count the beats in a full minute.

Your heart rate (pulse)

The normal pulse rate is about 70–80. Athletes and active sportsmen will have a slower rate, possibly down as low as 40. The pulse is a very sensitive barometer of the strength of the heart. When it begins to increase in strength it will develop a longer stroke for less effort, and will become slower, more regular and more efficient. When this has happened you will know that you really are able to build up reserves of power and energy and that you will be able to take in your stride running for a bus or leaping up stairs two at a time without extra demands on your heart or your lungs.

A safe heart rate

The heart, like everything else in the body, has its own range of rates of work. Its top rate is about 200 beats a minute, but this gets less with age, and deteriorates even more in those who are unfit. So, although you may feel perfectly fit in what you do at present, you may really be taxing an unfit heart and unfit lungs by putting additional strains upon them. This is how you identify your safety limit:

156

Subtract your age from 200.
Subtract another 40 if unfit.

So if you are a 50-year-old who is not fit, you will have subtracted 50 and 40, which tells you that your maximum safe pulse rate is 110. This level of 110 beats to the minute should not be exceeded during exercise, and strict observance of this formula will ensure that you will be working below three quarters of your heart's actual capacity, and this is safe. As you become fitter you can, of course, reduce the 'unfit penalty', within limits. You might start by reducing the 40 beat penalty one at a time. If you are in your 40s, or over, do not reduce it down to zero. To be on the safe side you should not reduce the penalty of 40 to less than 15. If you are over 50, do not reduce it below 20. If you are under 30 you can reduce the unfit penalty to zero and work with your own pulse rate.

Take your pulse rate at rest, eg when you are lying in bed, and let us say it is 70. Step up and down on one step of the stairs for two minutes. At the end you should not be breathless and you should be fully capable of holding a conversation with someone, and your pulse rate should come down to your normal rate of 70 within two minutes of stopping. If it does not and you are breathing hard, you are not fit. If you feel dizzy, or your chest hurts, or you get exceptionally breathless and cannot talk, you should see your family doctor and get your blood pressure checked. Whatever you do, start with warming up exercises, and build up gradually to a full exercise programme.

A fitness test

When we have not been exercising properly for some years, we have to condition ourselves by warming up before any kind of exercise. This warm-up period increases the body temperature, warms the muscles and gently stretches the tendons and joint ligaments thus preventing injury, stiffness or soreness. It also increases the heart activity and circulation slightly without undue strain.

Warm up first

1 *Arm stretch*
Stretch the arms above the head as high as possible. Bring them down to your side stretching forwards all the way down. Repeat 10 times. Next stretch from the top out sideways and down and up again via the front. Repeat 10 times.

Warm-up exercises

157

2 Trunk stretch
With hands on hips and feet slightly apart for balance, back straight and without bending forwards, tilt the trunk down 10 times to the right and 10 times to the left.

3 Back stretch
Sit on the floor and stretch the trunk forwards to grasp the toes, 10 times. Do these stretches slowly and do not push or force them. Flexibility, and the ability to grasp your toes, will come.

4 Abdominal stretch
Lie on the floor with legs straight and arms folded across the chest. Now raise the head, neck and back, slowly off the floor in an unfolding motion. When sitting up, let it all unroll slowly back again. If you can only get part of the way, do not worry. You will get fit. Ten times is average fitness, but do not overdo it. Keep the stretching sequences smooth and easy.

5 Leg stretch
Lie on the floor with your legs straight out and your arms by your sides. Now lift one leg up to the vertical, pointing the toe towards the ceiling. Repeat with the other leg, 10 times each. Now lift both legs together to the vertical, placing your hands under your buttocks for support, and stretch the legs over gently until your toes touch the floor behind your head. Come back to rest in an unrolling movement and repeat.

6 Chest stretch
Use the dining table for this exercise. Stand firmly, feet slightly apart for balance, at about two easy paces from the table with hands on the table edge. Now keeping the body straight, bend your arms until your chest touches the table, and then straighten the arms again. Five to 10 of these press ups is good, but do not overdo it.

7 Heart and lung strengthener
End the sequence with running on the spot. The higher you bring the knees, the more efficient this exercise is, but, if you have not done it before, just move gently for only a minute and then check your pulse rate at the end.

After a warming-up session always sit down and take your pulse. Two minutes later take it again, when it should have dropped back to your normal. As your work-outs become more taxing, the pulse may well stay high for two minutes. As you get fitter it will slow down sooner and you will need to take it at one and a half minutes, and then one minute, to

158

see the drop. You will know then that your heart has strengthened considerably.

If you are unfit

If you are unfit do only the warm-up exercises, followed by walking or swimming. Begin at an easy rhythmical, but slow pace, breathing deeply as you do them. If you have any apparatus such as an exercise bike or a rowing machine, bring them into your exercise routine at the end of the warm up. Increase both the time and the pressure gradually, watching your pulse rate at the end of each session. Aim for 15 minutes each morning and evening, or for a set time that you can keep to daily. This gradual build up is reconditioning and the weekends should be kept for longer walks further afield. When you have reconditioned yourself in this way, then you can join a club and build up strength, agility and energy on all their apparatus, or join the runners or joggers. But you must recondition first. Remember to allow a minimum of one month of this reconditioning for every year since you last exercised properly. There are far too many 'weekend athletes' who die of a heart attack from the sudden pressure on an unconditioned system.

Cooling down

Just as you need to give time to warming up, so you will need to give time to cooling down naturally. After exercising vigorously, gently ease off, slowing down but still moving until the breathing returns to normal and the body has cooled. Pull on a sweater, sit down and check your pulse rate, always keeping in mind your safety level of three quarters of your heart's maximum capacity.

What kind of exercise to strengthen the heart?

There are many different kinds of exercise and each has its devotees. There are isotonic and isometric exercises for building up strength in particular muscles. There are circuit training, weight lifting, running, jogging, and any number of ball games. For a long, fit, healthy life we have to pay most attention to the form of exercise that increases our breathing thereby strengthening the lungs, heart and circulation. The best for this are brisk walking interspersed with gentle running to vary the pace and the interest, and, best of all, swimming. Playing golf or gentle tennis is fine for interest in the open air, but is not 'conditioning'. Hard tennis, badminton and swimming, if you are concentrating on improving your speed, strength and stamina, is conditioning. Swimming is the one exercise that uses all your

159

muscles and increases your lung power as well. Cycling is good for the leg muscles and for the heart and circulation. Energetic squash and jogging should not be attempted until you are really fit, which your reconditioning warm-up exercises and brisk walking will do for you. Running up stairs will also recondition you. Working with your pulse rate as your guide, gradually increase the number of flights that you can run up at any one time.

Aerobic
exercises

The type of exercises recommended here are the type called aerobic, which simply means measuring vitality through increased oxygen consumption. If the exercises force you to breathe more deeply in order to perform them, then they are aerobic. But if they make such a demand that you are breathless and cannot talk, they are defeating the object of the exercise, and you are attempting too much too quickly. Build up slowly to fitness, and, again, remember that you have been a long time getting unfit.

Competitive and
non-competitive
sport

Both have their devotees and their merits. For stress proofing the system, we are concerned mainly with keeping a balance. If the main stress is on our mental abilities during the day, then we need to stimulate the physical and the emotional, and relax the intellectual function. In the same way, if we have a job where we have to be highly competitive all day, and then we play competitive sports, there is too much expenditure of effort. Effort puts high strain on the cardiovascular system (heart and circulation) and we could be in danger of pressing it too far. Our interest must be in strengthening it. So I would urge that if you have a highly competitive job and have to make continual effort in that, then find your physical outlet in uncompetitive activity such as walking.

Walk or jog?

Many people believe that walking does not constitute an 'exercise programme', and that to get fit one has to do something spectacular like running, jogging or playing squash. This is far from being the case. A comparative study was recently carried out on men aged 40–57. They were divided into two groups. One group jogged for 30 minutes, three days a week, while the other group walked at a brisk pace for 40 minutes, four days a week. The improvement to the walkers' fitness and health proved to be equal to that of the joggers. Studies like this are

160

important because for everyone over the age of 40, walking is much safer than jogging.

Walking, to be effective in strengthening the heart and circulation, must be regular and must be kept up for at least one hour three times a week or half an hour every day. A pace of three miles an hour is moderate. Four miles an hour is a fast pace that is demanding and may well prove too strenuous for people over 50, unless they are already fit. Three and a half miles an hour is possibly a good compromise. Brisk walking, as well as being pleasant and enjoyable, lowers the levels of carbon monoxide and nicotine in the circulation – a helpful piece of information for smokers who find it difficult to give up the habit. There is also evidence that narrowed areas in the coronary blood vessels can be opened up, thereby lessening the risk of heart disease. It also tones up the arteries rendering them less likely to furring up. Finally, the resting heart rate is decreased which indicates the strengthening of the heart and its circulation.

Walking to strengthen the heart

   Brisk walking clears away the biochemicals of stress and fatigue. It clears depression, dissipates anger and irritation, and by improving the blood supply to the brain naturally, heightens our thinking and problem-solving abilities. So walk the problems, the pressures and the effort away. It is better for the heart.

CHAPTER 12

Getting the physical balance right: food

People have talked more nonsense about food and how to slim 'safely' than about any other single health topic. Many have made themselves millionaires in the process, but in the process have increased the stress on our energy systems and left us irritable, fatigued and prey to every infection that comes along. And we are confused. We do not know whether to eat beans and nuts and give up meat ('I thought meat was good for you for its iron?'); whether to eat brown bread or white ('Some people say that the brown is just white bread dyed and it's the same thing really.'); whether to give up all dairy produce ('My mother used to say it was good for you, she'd make us drink milk and put butter on our vegetables for goodness.'), and now we hear that we should not drink coffee because it has got caffeine in it. But so has tea and cocoa and Coca Cola, so what do we drink? We have been told to diet to get weight off and now we hear that dieting makes you fat so what *do* we do?

You eat a little of everything is the answer: meat, vegetables, fruit, eggs, butter, milk, tea, coffee – everything in moderation. Do not overdo any one thing. Coffee, of course, has caffeine in it which stimulates the system, so do tea and cocoa to a slightly lesser extent.

Three cups of coffee a day is fine and so, sometimes, is more, but some people in offices are drinking coffee continuously from the coffee machines at work and totting up as many as seven or eight cups a day plus what they drink at home, and this is too much.

So let us dispel a few of the myths about food; say how we use energy during the day and how much we need; and then we can work out for ourselves what kind of diet is best for us to either lose weight or to put on weight. We will take some of the myths first.

Dispelling a few myths about food

1 *'The perfect slimming diet.'*
There is no such thing. Every diet has its merits and with each one you will first lose fluid and so drop a few pounds, then the tissue not needed by the body will go and if you starve enthusiastically the body will cling on to its reserves believing that it is in a famine situation and has to conserve its essential fats, so you will come to the plateau so well known to all dieters. At this point one usually gives up or decides to stay at that weight. The body, believing that the famine is over once food is taken again, builds up its reserves ready for the next famine. So on go the pounds again although you eat very little. There is only one way to control weight and that is the physiologically balanced way of burning up food by oxygen to produce energy. If you eat a well-balanced diet, the body knows that it will not be starved. Then you take in plenty of oxygen through movement and activity to burn it all up and produce energy. You become fit, vigorous and energetic, able to step up your activities which again burns up the food, producing yet more energy. It really is not difficult if we work with the body. It is built for the different times of plenty and famine and has highly complex storage systems. We have to work with these, not against them, if we want to trim the figure.

2 *'Bran is essential to a healthy diet.'*
Bran has no food content. It is useful, in the same way as cabbage stalks and other fibre are, to give one's stool bulk and make elimination easier and more complete. It does not help 'slimming', it is not 'healthy', it is not good for you. It may actually be harmful if you eat bran to the exclusion of a balanced diet and different types of fibre. Fibre is the waste or residue from meat, fruits, vegetables and whole grain cereals, and it is these we need; the residue will then take care of itself.

3 *'You do not need vitamins if you have a balanced diet.'* Most writers on nutrition would agree with this, but they should add, 'If we eat plenty of citrus fruit every day and a salad; shop for fresh vegetables daily and eat at least two servings of these a day; lead lives free from worry and anxiety and eat whole grain breads and cereals.' We have to face the fact that we usually shop only once a week and the vegetables will probably have been stored in the shop and stored in our pantry and so will have lost most of their vitamin C by the time we cook them. They will lose the rest

163

in cooking and keeping hot. Many of us have a quick sandwich lunch making do with the kind of bread they have in the shop. We have not the time to sit and eat a salad or a pound or two of vegetables even if we had the inclination, so we are not going to have sufficient vitamin C in the diet nor enough of the vitamin B complex. Both the vitamin B complex and vitamin C are released with the stress chemicals. Their exact function in stress is not known but we do know that when these vitamins are taken in addition to the diet the general health improves quite remarkably. So if you are handling crises in your life do take vitamin B complex and vitamin C. You will need the one-gramme, effervescent vitamin C tablets which you can drop in water. These are available at any good chemist, but the full vitamin B group tablets (B complex meaning every B vitamin included) are not. You will need to go to a health food store for these.

4 *'You do not lose weight by exercising.'*
Yes you do. Running up stairs uses 20 calories a minute. True, it takes 3,500 calories to burn off one pound in weight, but a half hour's walk to work or to the station and back at a moderate pace of three miles an hour will lose you three pounds a month just by walking. Walk fast, four miles an hour, and use the stairs instead of lifts and you can double it. But more than this, the effects of this naturally speeded up body and brain function last long after you have stopped, so the actual loss of fat is higher. There is a gain in energy through the increased oxygen intake and you will be losing fat and not lean muscle if you are active. The body only gets rid of what it is not using.

Can we rely on appetite as a guide to a balanced diet? Yes, we can. If everything is laid out on tables in front of us and all we have to do is put them on a plate we tend to choose a balanced selection of foods. Research shows that after we have gone for things we have not had for some time, like strawberries and cream, even children will pick from the different dishes and give themselves a good, mixed diet. The snag is that we never do have everything prepared and laid out for us in this way. So are there any golden rules for ensuring that we do have a balanced diet in the home? Yes there are a few.

Guide lines to a good diet

1 Know your foods by groups and choose a little of every group at every meal. The body needs 10 essential amino

164

acids from the proteins, about 20 different minerals and thirteen vitamins in order to ensure that it has the basic chemicals to make up everything it needs for building tissues, making red blood cells, making antibodies and enzymes and for all its varied work. So we need a mixed diet.

2   Try to shop twice a week for vegetables so that they are fresh, and have four or five different kinds (in very small helpings, of course) at the main meal of the day.

3   Try to have a salad at lunch. If you have a sandwich, have a salad sandwich and take a piece of fruit or a tomato to have with it.

4   We rely upon vegetables to get those 20 or so minerals so really pile them in. If you have fish and chips, add peas or tomatoes. If you have eggs and bacon, add tomatoes or mushrooms. Always add a vegetable to whatever you eat and you will have a balance.

5   Try to grow your own vegetables. If necessary, beg or borrow an allotment or a piece of a neighbour's garden. It is better to know that chemical sprays are not being applied to your food. Failing this, try to find vegetables which have been grown organically without chemical fertilisers.

6   Have fruit instead of a pudding, or as well as, if you have hungry teenagers to feed. The golden rule is to mix a lot of different things. So let us say, for example, that you buy marrow, runner beans, celery and carrots. Cook a very little of them for each meal instead of just one large helping of one of them, and serve in small dishes. You will find that, if given the choice, the family will help themselves to a good, mixed diet. Let your body have the basic chemicals it needs and you will not be tired and lethargic. The body can only make its various chemical chains from what you put into it – give it the variety it needs.

What foods should I eat?

A little of everything. Most foods contain complex mixtures of chemicals and we need those mixtures. Everything (except sugar) is a mixture of water, proteins, carbohydrates, lipids, vitamins, minerals and fibre. As we have said, we need about 20 minerals and about 30 vitamins to be really fit, vigorous and energetic. You will know, of course, that some foods are classed as proteins and others as carbohydrates, but this can be misleading. Carbohydrates contain mainly carbon, hydrogen and oxygen; proteins contain carbon, hydrogen and oxygen with the addition of other chemicals such as sulphur and phosphorus.

165

When the body has split the proteins down into its basic building blocks (amino acids) and taken what it needs from these for its tissues, the rest – about 20 per cent carbon, hydrogen and oxygen – can be used to supply energy in the same way as carbohydrates. So it is perhaps easier for most of us to group the different foodstuffs and aim to eat a little from each group at every meal to be sure that we get the full chemical mixtures which the body and brain need.

The five basic groups of food

1 Dairy produce.
2 Meat, fish, eggs and poultry.
3 Vegetables.
4 Fruit.
5 Breads and cereals.

Group 1: dairy produce

These are milk and all milk products, like soups with dried milk, drinks like milk shakes, desserts like custards, rice puddings, sauces made with milk, cheese, butter and ice-cream. From this group you obtain calcium – our main supply –, riboflavin, protein and vitamins A and D. Milk contains all the nutrients needed for the young child (particularly its own mother's milk), so it is rich in nearly all the nutrients – fat, carbohydrate, protein and most of the vitamins and minerals, particularly calcium, phosphorus and potassium. It lacks only vitamin C and is short in vitamin D, iron and copper. It is a valuable food for children. Butter and cream supply vitamins A and D as well as fat. So cream should be eliminated altogether if you want to lose weight, and butter kept to a minimum. Skimmed milk and curd or cottage cheese could be substituted for the full-fat variety, but make sure that you get vitamins A and D in your cereals as they are lost from skimmed milk.

Group 2: meat, fish, poultry, eggs

This is the protein group and also includes beans (dried). From this group you get protein, iron – especially from liver, eggs and meat, vitamins A and B, thiamine – especially from pork thiamine and iron – from peas and dried beans and nuts.

Eggs are rich in protein and fats and have little carbohydrate. They contain nearly all the vitamins and minerals except calcium. Eggs and milk together for invalids or children are therefore rich in practically all of the essentials. Meat is rich in iron and some of the B vitamins – riboflavin, nicotinic acid and B12 – whereas liver is rich in

166

all vitamins. This group is not high in calcium unless whitebait, sardines and other whole fish, including the bones, are eaten. Cut off all fat from meat and aim to eat eggs and meat no more than three times a week, or eat only in small amounts.

Most root vegetables are high in carbohydrate and fibre but low in vitamins, except carrots which have vitamin A. Leafy vegetables are rich in protein and high in vitamins and minerals. They have vitamins of the B group, particularly folic acid, riboflavin and nicotinic acid, iron, calcium and potassium. Vitamin C is high but is lost in storage and cooking, as it is water soluble, ie leaks out in water. There is increasing evidence that people who eat plenty of fresh vegetables do not get stomach cancer. Cabbage, brussel sprouts, broccoli, cauliflower, spinach and celery all aid the making of protective enzymes against cancer. This has led to the interest in fresh vegetables in the treatment of patients with cancer. *Group 3: vegetables*

Vegetables lose their vitamins quickly when stored. Only buy them from shops where you know they are fresh, ie with a good turnover of produce. Do not buy more than you need for two days, and, if you can, cut them up very small and stir fry them in very little sunflower oil for only a minute or two. Have two or more servings of vegetables a day. From this group we obtain all minerals – our main source, vitamin A – in dark green leafy vegetables and carrots, vitamin B – in dark green leafy vegetables, vitamin C in raw vegetables and salads, and also in carrots, leeks, parsnips, turnips and beetroot, calcium and iron in leeks.

Fruits are high in water content and in carbohydrate; they are low in fat and protein and many are rich in vitamin C, eg blackcurrants, oranges, lemons, grapefruit, limes and tomatoes. As with vegetables, we should have two servings or more of fruit every day. At least one of these should be citrus or tomatoes for our vitamin C. Fruit juices, unless pure, are probably not from fruit at all. Frozen fruits, like vegetables, are useful when fresh are not in season. From these we get vitamin C – our main source. *Group 4: fruits*

This group contains all the breads, the breakfast cereals, the uncooked cereals like rice, spaghetti, noodles, macaroni and all the pastas. It also includes all those products made with flour and yeast like cakes and biscuits. Cereals *Group 5: breads and cereals* are the major source of food for all the peoples of the earth. Some have rice, others spaghetti, others maize or cassava or wheat to which they add small pieces of meat, fish and vegetables. All contain protein, some fat, some carbohydrate. They contain most vitamins of the B group and vitamin E. However, most of them are lost in milling and processing. So white flour and white rice are nutritionally poor. Therefore, our bread, which should be our staple diet, is nutritionally poor if it is white. From this group we get thiamine, riboflavin, niacin and iron.

If we eat 'real' bread made from stone-ground flour, the original wheatgerm and all the minerals and the vitamin B complex will still be there.

The correct amounts of these groups for a balanced diet are:

Group 1	Some daily, half pint skimmed milk if 'slimming'. Some cheese for the calcium.
Group 2	One serving of meat only. Try to alternate with poultry and fish or eggs, cutting down on the meat, possibly to three times a week.
Group 3	At least two servings daily. If you had only one vegetable at lunchtime or a salad, have a main meal of vegetables in the evening.
Group 4	At least two serving of these a day. Eat all the fruits in season.
Group 5	Eat only whole grain from stone-ground flour if possible, you will find it difficult to eat more than two slices at a time. Cut out cakes and biscuits and the pastas if you are overweight.

We need to take in some foods together so that the body gets a balance and can make all the chemicals it needs from those we give it. We must eat breakfast so that the chemical work of the body can proceed and we should take in from Groups 1, 2, 4 and 5. Orange juice, cereal and milk and an egg or a piece of cheese like Edam or cottage cheese (low in fat) and a slice of wholegrain bread will make sure that the body has the chemicals it needs and we will remain alert, vigorous and energetic for the morning. At lunchtime and at the evening meal we need to take from every group.

168

1   Buy some brown rice and try it in risotto dishes. It is nutty in flavour and full of the B vitamins needed for stress proofing. It will need longer cooking than white rice. You will like the flavour and it is good with savoury dishes.

2   Have at least two vegetable meals a week and use many different vegetables together at other meals to make sure that you receive your full supply of minerals.

3   Have at least one salad dish twice a week full of vitamin C in the winter. A good one is the Waldorf salad which has oranges, grapefruit and grapes surrounding the basic salad of apple and celery with walnuts. Toppings for salads to make them different and more nutritious are grilled chopped bacon, toasted garlic bread crumbed and sprinkled over the top, blue cheese dressing, chopped hard-boiled egg, chopped walnuts or other nuts.

4   Buy a loaf of bread made with 100 per cent stone-ground flour and try it. It has a satisfying bite to it and is packed full of vitamins. It is very good toasted.

5   Grill all meat, fish and bacon instead of frying. This cuts down the fat content and cuts out fat for frying.

6   Buy and use sunflower oil for cooking and use only a little just to prevent sticking, unless deep frying. This oil is tasteless and gets crisp results. It can be used for salads as well.

7   Use small amounts of meat for flavouring with plenty of vegetables in casseroles and stews.

8   Eat more fish, poultry and liver.

9   Eat some fruit at every meal.

10   Use more dried beans and pulses of all kinds in cooking for cheap, highly nutritious, protein and vitamin meals. Beans lower the cholesterol in the blood and like the brassicas (cabbage, sprouts, etc) protect against cancer.

11   Eat wholemeal breakfast cereals.

12   Cut out all bought sugar from the diet. Try sweetening with honey instead.

13   Cut down on processed food as much as possible in order to reduce the intake of the chemicals used in the preservation and colouring of the food.

Fairly easily, if we go by how our system works, how it stores and how it uses energy. We take in food which is burned up in the presence of oxygen which gives us our energy. We use a lot of energy in living. If we use up most of what we take in there will be little to store. The object of *How can we get this slimming business straight?*

taking weight off is to burn up some of our stored fat. So far this is straightforward. Bodies are misers when food is scarce. Our bodies are very wise. They will learn to make do with a very frugal diet if they think there is a famine on, ie that no food is coming their way. So they will stop burning up food to give us energy and cling on to their stores like an old miser hoarding every penny as he sees his stocks running low. So, follow the golden rule of taking in a little of everything, including wholemeal bread (more satisfying in small doses) and potatoes, while putting the emphasis on lots of different vegetables for your minerals. The body will see that there is no shortage of food and will not hoard its tissues.

Ensure the tissue you lose is fat

The body is made up of many different kinds of tissue, but when we are slimming we are interested in losing only one kind, and that is fat. The body is interested in keeping the tissues that it needs, eg muscular, lean tissue for athletes and all active people, and fat for its stores for energy and the stress response in times of hazard, change and additional demand. So if you are not highly active, what will the body give up first? The lean tissue and not the reserve stores of fat. So, again, go with your own function. You have already signalled that there is plenty of food so the body can cut down its hoarding. Now you have to signal that you need your lean, muscular tissue. The only way to do that is to start to use it. Now you are all set to use the equation of how much you have to take in in order to have the energy necessary to do everything you need to do, and at the same time get the body to burn up some of its fat.

Keep all the energy you need

We measure the energy value of food, and the energy that we use, in terms of calories. Our food is burned up to release all the different chemicals we need for the functioning of the body and brain, to keep us warm, and to provide energy. The average office worker, or any one in a sedentary occupation, needs about 2,500 calories a day. If you think of a steam engine, it consumes energy (coal) when it is standing in the station, just as we do when we are sitting down. When the engine starts to move it consumes more energy and the faster it moves, or the greater its load, the more fuel it uses. Just like us, the more we do and the more weight we carry, the more fuel we use.

170

Yes, the body and brain are working throughout our lives, and therefore using up energy all the time.

	calories used per minute
Sleeping	1.1
Washing and dressing (if fast)	3.0
Walking to work (if fast)	5.2
Driving to work	2.8
Sitting	1.5
Sitting and writing	2.0
Standing	1.56
Light domestic work	3.0
Gardening	4.8
Swimming	14.0

You will be able to add up what you do, and if you move quickly, how many calories you use. Let us suppose your day is divided up as follows.

		calories used
Sleep	8 hours	528
Washing and dressing	½ hour	90
Walking	1 hour	312
Sitting	3 hours	270
Sitting and writing	1½ hours	240
Driving to work	1 hour	168
Standing activities	4 hours	456
Light sedentary	4 hours	360
Light domestic	1 hour	180
	Total	2604

If you sit for more than this, or do not do the hour of walking, you can clearly see that, with an average daily intake of 2,600 calories, you are inevitably going to get fatter.

So, step up the movement. You will soon be into that smaller suit or dress, and feeling trim, fit, and highly energetic.

1 Aim for a long, slow reorganisation in your lifestyle: not a 'crash course' diet. Change your eating habits to lots of vegetables and your sedentary habits to lots of walking, and you will probably have to do nothing else.
2 Cut out all cakes, biscuits and sugar, but nothing else.

171

3 Do take vitamins and extra minerals if you are not eating three or four vegetables each day.
4 Only weigh yourself once a week.
5 Calculate your energy expenditure, and increase it.
6 Buy a pocket book of the calorie values of foods and only eat a little of the very high group such as cream.

To increase your weight

Keep to the balance suggested in the five main groups, but you do not have to cut out the full cream or the cakes and biscuits. It is not a good idea to increase your sugar intake. Sugar has no food value at all. Increase the helpings of the five main groups, and have sauces with your vegetables: cheese sauce with cauliflower or white sauce with marrow etc. Mixtures of fat and flour stay longer in the stomach, and are more satisfying. Have soups with toast or croutons before your two main meals. Have a mid-morning snack and another in the afternoon. Have milk shakes and hot chocolate instead of coffee. Sit over your meals for as long as possible and relax after them for about half an hour. If you are unduly anxious – and thin underweight people often are – read Chapter 14 on handling anxiety.

CHAPTER 13

Getting the emotional balance right: depression

Everyone becomes depressed from time to time. Whether we live in a palace, a high-rise flat, in a town or on a beautiful Hebridean island, we are all vulnerable to the blues. The only things which seem to make a difference are being a woman, (women are twice as likely to suffer the blues as men), being a church-goer (they are a third less likely to suffer than the non church-goers) and having plenty of friends. If we have friends with whom to share our problems we are far less likely to suffer from the more serious kinds of depression.

How much depression is there?

This is difficult to estimate because many depressed people do not know that they are suffering from depression, and many of those who do know do not realise that it is a treatable illness, and so do not 'worry the doctor' with it. So it is difficult to estimate. In the United States, it is acknowledged to be a major health problem affecting about 15 per cent of the population. Their suicide rate is very high, running at about 30,000 every year and attempted suicides are numbered in hundreds of thousands. Suicide is, unfortunately, all too common an ending to the more serious type of depression known as endogenous, luckily not the most prevalent of the depressive illnesses.

In Britain, well over half of all patients are seen by GPs for anxiety and depression, but only about five per cent of people with symptoms of anxiety or depression actually go to their doctors. So it is thought that the problem is large. The difficulty of arriving at figures is connected with the problem of identifying the illness. Depressed people are often thought by others to be 'in a mood', 'sulking', or even 'bloody minded' and are told to 'cheer up', 'snap out of it', or to 'stop going round like a wet week'. They themselves are unable to say, 'I'm ill with a depressive illness.' They

173

are only aware of a cloud of gloom, ranging from sadness to abject despair. They feel alone, although they may be surrounded by family, and life appears to be utterly meaningless. It is essential to recognise depression, particularly the more serious type, and this chapter will help you to do this.

How many kinds of depression are there?

There are several. Some are part of our normal swings of mood. We have ups when we feel we could climb Everest, win a beauty contest or conquer the world, and we have downs when nothing seems to go right. These I call, having a down day and having a fit of the blues.

The down day is a very short spell of feeling down in the doldrums. It can be triggered off by something quite simple like oversleeping yet again, and is just as quickly dispelled by something nice happening to us. A cheerful 'good morning' from a neighbour can make the spirits soar again.

A fit of the blues lasts longer, perhaps two or three days, and may occur simply because the body is fighting some infection and is not doing too well in the battle. We, of course, are not conscious of this, we only know that we feel low and 'under par'. It may also occur through a rebuff, through a row with a close friend, or work may get on top of us and we feel, temporarily, that life is all work and no play. Sooner or later, though, the up-swings come, our spirits lift and we forget that we have ever felt blue.

The real depressions

There are the real depressions, though, which are illnesses, and they need recognising and treating. They are of two main types: re-active depression and endogenous depression.

Re-active depression

This is triggered off by things which cause us distress. It might be the loss of our job, of our love, or of our standing in the community. It could be failure to succeed at things which are important to us. It is also sometimes triggered off by our failure to do our best. For example, many GPs now suffer from depression through the sheer inability to practise really good medicine because of their workload. People in all walks of life suffer from this pressure of time and overload of work, while at the other end of the scale those who have lost their jobs suffer from depression through sheer frustration and hopelessness. Re-active depression, as its name implies, is depression caused by our reaction to

174

these highly stressful events in our lives. It is the most common of the depressive illnesses.

This is a more rare type of depressive illness and is very much more to do with our biochemistry. It is called endogenous from the word 'endo' meaning inside. It can be serious and the feeling of black despair in these cases carries with it a high risk of suicide. In the most severe cases it is as if there is a heavy damp blanket cutting out the sun, the warmth, and all feeling. The ability to love, to laugh, to feel interest in, to communicate, to enjoy food, to feel moved by anything, all goes. It is as if all information about the outside world has stopped. This is in fact what happens.

Endogenous depression

It is now known that some of the brain chemicals which are involved in transmitting information between one nerve cell and another (the neurotransmitters) are altered in this type of depression. Their production is low. This, of course, affects all our function; the brain rhythms in sleep are altered, all sexual drive usually stops, appetite for food goes and the storage of food is altered and weight often drops alarmingly. If there is an excess of production, which can happen, then mania, the opposite of depression, occurs. People suffering from both swings are termed manic-depressives. This is now a condition easily treatable by Lithium Salts and your GP can easily arrange this. As endogenous depression is such a tragic condition, it is well worth while knowing how to recognise it.

Information from outside does not reach us

The following signs differentiate this type of depression from the more common re-active depression.

Recognising endogenous (primary) depression

1 It may occur suddenly 'out of the blue'.
2 There is no apparent cause for it.
3 There may be a family history of a like condition: manic-depression, mania or hypomania or depression.
4 It can be long-lasting – three to nine months.
5 It has a tendency to recur, so patients have usually had one or more bouts of depression in their lives, again for no apparent cause.
6 Suicide is a real danger in a serious attack when one feels utterly hopeless.

How depressed are you?   Answer each statement with the reply 'True' or 'False'.

1   I feel low.
2   I wake early in the morning drenched with sweat.
3   I feel really miserable all day.
4   I dread waking – there is nothing to get up for.
5   I burst into tears for just no reason.
6   I've no appetite at all so I don't eat.
7   I feel scared and panicky if I have to do anything.
8   I feel helpless and unable to deal with life any more.
9   I lose my temper and snap at people.
10 I've got this grey cloud settled all around me.
11 The only time I'm roused is when friends come in.
12 I've lost all interest in sex and I had a normally strong drive.
13 The only enjoyment is my children, when they come to see me I perk up.
14 I find it impossible to smile, to laugh and to have fun any more.
15 I feel ugly and a terrible mess.
16 I don't care what I look like any more.
17 I suffer from headaches and pains in my joints.
18 I have vivid dreams and wake a lot and I used to be a very heavy sleeper.
19 I'm all right at work if things are happening all the time.
20 I really feel like ending it all – what is the future?
21 I know what caused all this but I can't get out of it by myself.
22 I don't know why I'm like this, there's no reason for it.
23 I don't think anyone can help me.
24 I don't really feel anything; it's as if time has stopped still.

If you have answered 'true' to statements 1, 3, 5, 9, 11, 15, 19 and 21 you probably have a mild re-active depression and you can come out of it and stay up with the help of this Chapter.

If you have answered 'true' to statements 2, 3, 4, 5, 7, 9, 11, 13, 14, 15, 16, 17, 18, 21 and 23 you have a re-active depression from some deep distress. The section on handling depression will help you, but in addition you will also need to carry out the relaxation techniques in Chapter 8.

176

Find a friend to help you and do them together.

If you have answered 'true' to the statements with even numbers your depression is likely to be mainly endogenous. Luckily, today there are ways of replacing the shortage of chemicals produced in the system and one or other of the many new anti-depressant drugs on the market will help you and you will need only one or two weeks on them. Do go and talk it over with your GP because you can get back to normal quickly with the right one. Your GP may find it helpful if you take this quiz and your answers along with you.

Children may suffer from depression for two main reasons. The first is because of a sense of failure. They may feel unable to compete with a successful brother or sister; unable to get a higher place in their class no matter how hard they try; unable to obtain the full love and attention of a parent. The second reason is loss. Loss of an adored pet, a loved grandparent, or the loss of one parent from the home. The finality of death, although causing grief, is in the long run less damaging for a later history of depression than loss through a parent walking out and leaving the child behind. This may be the cause of a mild endogenous depression at adolescence if things go badly emotionally when the biochemistry is changing.

Depression affects all ages

Adolescents become alternately depressed and elated very quickly. Their changing body chemistry throws their emotional stability off balance and they may feel in the depths of despair over something quite trivial which would not normally affect them. Earlier emotional upsets may re-occur at this time and may lead to depression and sadness or anger, rebellion and a withdrawal from parents.

For women, depression may occur as the body chemistry changes before a period, after the birth of a baby and again at the change of life when childbearing comes to an end. The feeling of failure is also a prime trigger for depression. The failure of not being able to achieve a satisfying sexual life or a longed-for child or a successful career for which one previously trained, are prime examples. Similarly, failure to achieve success as a wife and mother can cause depression, particularly if one's children turn to glue sniffing, drugs, or socially unacceptable behaviour.

For men, depression can occur at any age, but is more likely as part of the mid-life blues: the 'What have I achieved' stage between 40 and 50.

177

Handling depression

Although the normal downs and the blues will come and go they need looking after, because at difficult and trying times, and we all have them, it is easy for those natural downs to depress our mood, stay longer than they should and cause us to slide into a real depression.

The physical sphere

The downs and the blues can occur when our systems are fighting infections, mopping up alien cells, dealing with alcohol, nicotine and other drugs and unwanted chemicals which we take in with food and drink. Therefore we can help our systems by:

1   Keeping the food we take in as pure and uncontaminated as possible.

2   Leaving a week or two in between parties and entertaining when we are likely to eat, drink and smoke more than usual.

3   Taking one gramme daily of vitamin C if feeling low. This is the anti-infective vitamin and it helps the body to fight infections.

4   Taking the vitamin B complex, including B12. If you cannot get vitamin B complex with B12 (look at the contents carefully – B12 is called Cytocon), buy it separately but take all the B vitamins together as we need a balance of all of them in the body.

5   Living a well balanced lifestyle. See Chapter 10.

The emotional sphere

Everyone has their own spirit lifters. Mine are music and walking in woods. I really need loud music most of the day when feeling stressed or down, preferably piano concertos. These lifters are associated with emotional satisfaction at critical ages and each us will have different ones.

You will have your own emotional lifts and it is worth thinking them out and then planning to have access to them whenever you feel the need. They not only lift you from depression but can actually save your life. Charles, a dress designer of 42 years of age, had cancer which he was told was terminal. As there was really nothing the hospital could do for him he discharged himself. He had heard that someone had cured themselves with laughter and laughter was important to him. So he bought a video and tapes of the funniest films he could find. He loved the children's cartoon characters like Donald Duck, really funny farces and *Punch*. He armed himself with all the funnies he could find on film and in books and comics and he literally laughed himself back to life.

178

You need understanding friends; friends who are sympathetic and will listen and talk with you about your problems. It is quite true that a problem shared is a problem halved. This is not always easy. The difficulty in bereavement, for example, as opposed to loss of love in a divorce or separation, is that friends are very diffident and do not know whether it helps to say nothing or to talk about the deceased. It really does help to talk about him or her in order for the partner to come to terms with the finality of the situation. Only then can one begin to think of them as people we have loved rather than as extensions of the self and therefore still here.

The social sphere

We need to develop friendships with all age groups, young and old, and widely spread in the community.

Remember, we said in the beginning that widespread friendships saved one from the deeper depressions as did also going to church. The churchgoers have the support of a spiritual belief and the social support of being a member of the 'family' of the church.

This will help all types of depression, endogenous as well as re-active. We think quite differently when we are depressed, have you noticed? 'It's no use,' 'I can't do . . .,' 'It won't work,' 'It's no earthly use trying that.' It is as if we have the record of positives and negatives in our brain and the needle is stuck in the negative. Analyse your thought patterns when you are depressed and you will discover that:

The thinking or cognitive sphere

1 They are firmly fixed on yourself.
2 They are only negative.
3 They only take a despondent view of the future. Everything is 'I can't,' 'It's no use.'

Now there are not very many things that we cannot do compared with everything that we can. As for the future, history has shown that all the gloomy forecasts have been wrong. The great plague did not wipe us all out. Hitler did not invade and overrun us. The world did not end as forecast and 1984 was not too terrible. When you are down it is the time to inject a little rationality into your thought patterns and start to change them.

Lift these thoughts out of their rut

Here is what you do every time you have the negative thoughts 'I can't,' 'It's no use.' You write it down and

179

change it into a positive one. Geoffrey was made redundant from a management job at 54 and depression hit him hard. He said 'It's no use' applying for another job, 'I'm too old'. 'What about trying for local firms?' he was asked. 'That's hopeless, I'm too old, too experienced for them and anyhow the pay wouldn't be any good.' What is the positive side of this? The local firms will employ him. Here is an experienced senior executive and many a local firm would consider themselves very fortunate in getting this level of expertise which would not have happened except for the recession. Certainly the pay will be lower but what are the positive gains? The positive aspects are the gain of two hours a day from travelling and the economic saving of the rail fare. More time for the family, for hobbies and for time to devote to thinking about starting a private enterprise later. And so it proved to be.

Choose to feel happier

So write down these negative thoughts and then write out the positive side of them. Every morning when you wake up you have two choices, one to feel sad, the other to feel happier. Think about it and then choose to feel happier. Think, 'I have chosen to feel happier today.' Now, what will help it to become possible? The way you look, what you wear and how you move.

Colour is important in depression. Decide to wear a colour that lifts you; a red suit, a crimson tie. Think about what you will wear and get out of bed. Getting out of bed is the worst hurdle over. Now attack the day positively. You are up and on your feet. Our thoughts determine to a great extent the way we feel. If we feel life is a drag we sag, our shoulders droop, the backbone sags, the tummy sticks out and we walk heavily and look (and feel) 100 years old. So walk over to the record player, put on a record you like, loudly, because it has to penetrate that grey blanket.

Now go to the mirror, stand up straight, tuck your bottom under and straighten the back. Feel as if there is a cord from the bottom of your spine to the top of your head and it is being pulled straight up to the ceiling. Comb your hair – it will still look lank at this stage, take no notice of this yet – and then smile. You will notice how the facial muscles lift. Now let the smile reach your eyes, listen to the music and let it reach you. Smile again into the mirror. Notice the lift to the body. You will have stopped sagging and you will have got a little life into the face. You are beginning to look more like yourself: like the child who was

180

cherished, the woman who was loved. You still have those qualities to inspire love and deep affection. Take them out and shine them up; you need them now. Look at your face again, smile and notice the immediate lift. Soon you will feel a little of this lift.

The positive thoughts and feelings to aim for are the opposite of the depressed thoughts. At present you feel hopeless. *Hope*. You know that this period will pass even if it lasts for months – it will eventually go *even if you do nothing*. So know that it will pass. We want it to go quickly though and you can help this. Now that you know that you will get better, begin to experience exactly how you feel. To start with, you will probably feel numb, so we have to work on that and get the emotional centres to work again. First tell the family that you know now that this will pass and that the very knowledge has made you feel a little lighter in spirit and ask them to help you to keep this lift however small, and help you increase it tomorrow. Now start to get those emotional centres working. Look at the garden, the flowers, the trees. This used to give you pleasure. How did you feel then? Try to recapture the feeling. Listen to the birds singing. This used to lift you. How did you feel? It was a warm glow, wasn't it? A feeling that all is right with the world. Try to recapture it now. Get out your favourite object: a toy, a picture, a record: something which used to give you pleasure and look and listen and think what the 'pleasure feeling' was like.

It will pass

The positive approaches will help you to begin to lift the gloom. Remember the three things to do:

1   Write down every negative thought and change it to a positive one.
2   Actively alter your appearance. Banish the sad slouch and regain your former lift and smile every time you pass the mirror. It will eventually reach your eyes and they will light up again.
3   Actively search for the happy emotions which you used to associate with the things you like. Warmth, affection, happiness and caring will come back as the emotional centres are stimulated and the depression will lift. In our true human way, you will soon have forgotten that you ever suffered from depression.

CHAPTER 14

Getting the emotional balance right: anxiety

Our emotions – love, hate, fear, anger – all serve a purpose in our lives. Because we are gregarious and need people, we have love, from the warmth of caring for our friends to the burning desire which ensures the continuation of our species. Because we are innately curious and so explore our world we have the emotion of fear which saves us from leaping off cliffs, swimming in shark-infested waters or walking through blazing forests. Because we have enemies we have anger and rage which gives us strength and energy to fight and overcome them.

A signal to act

Anxiety also serves a purpose. It is a signal to us that we have a hidden conflict or problem which needs dealing with. It is saying, in effect, 'You are throwing your emotional balance out and disturbing your peace of mind; deal with it. Plan that talk, speech, chapter, report, budget or whatever is hanging over you, in your diary now. Organise the time to do it and forget it.' Or, 'Your mother-in-law is destroying your marriage – assert yourself now.' In other words, it should be a signal for action, not left to fester into a state of anxiety. One is natural, normal and healthy: the other is an illness which needs treating. But as with depression there are many stages in between.

The everyday worries which we all face are not serious unless we allow them to accumulate and overwhelm us. Then in some people the unresolved conflicts can lead to more serious conditions called 'anxiety states' which are dangerous to health.

The stages of anxiety

Very few of us can remain carefree throughout life today. Most of us have problems, worries and cares to deal with. The worried and anxious personalities among us may, if they do not resolve their problems, end up with a mild anxiety state. It is estimated that about 10 per cent of the

182

population suffer from this illness and about half of that number will suffer a severe form of it. A few, believed to be well below 5 per cent of the population, will have so many unresolved conflicts that they have a nervous breakdown. This is no more really than the body saying to us, 'Enough is enough, I'm now taking a rest and getting myself back to normal.' The body is so much wiser than we are. But we knowledgeable ones are now going to be wise and stop the anxieties at the 'normal' stage. So let us look at these normal anxieties next.

A multitude of things. The full in-tray which no matter how fast we work is still over-flowing at the end of the day – every day. The letter from the bank manager, the income tax demand and our mortgage repayments which go up and up. Worrying events make us anxious. A small child running a high temperature, a member of the family unaccountably late home or a return to find the house burgled. Fears make us anxious. The fear of failure, of losing our job, of an incurable illness, or dying. Reality can also make us anxious. The realisation that at 45 we are now no longer likely to achieve the bright promises of our youth.

What makes us anxious?

These are the normal everyday anxieties which most of us in the Western industrial world battle with every day of our lives. In addition, having the world news of tragedies, disasters and frank terrorism brought into our homes daily in all the media adds to our anxieties and may well account for many of our moments of pessimism, gloom and despair which descend upon us out of the blue.

Anxiety only becomes serious when it is more than a passing phase, when it takes us over, producing an anxiety state which then affects our thinking, our feeling and our behaviour. At this point and in these states, loving husbands and wives can walk out and leave the family; parents can batter their children and each other and normal caring people can go berserk with disastrous consequences. These are the rarer tragedies from very severe anxiety states and, of course, they catch the attention of the press. But because they have such tragic consequences it is important to be able to recognise some of the signs.

When it becomes serious

It can be seen in the tense strained face and in every movement which instead of being smooth, flowing and co-ordinated becomes jerky, awkward and almost as if one

What are the signs of serious anxiety state

183

is a poorly controlled puppet. The voice is also a give away. It is high pitched and strained, and the words come tumbling out in rapid succession almost staccato fashion. The individual can be fretful, irritable, apprehensive and fearful by turns and there is a restlessness which prevents rest and relaxation. With such a pattern of high, jumpy and jerky activity, energy levels can go down suddenly and lead to exhaustion.

What can trigger an anxiety state? Many things. Anxiety is cumulative so there could be an underlying fear of redundancy, of failure or a lack of self-confidence. Then tensions can mount during the day at work, be added to in the fracas of the rush-hour and be compounded if there are serious problems in the home. All this could tip one over into an anxiety state, mild or severe.

Other things which can act as triggers are accidents, illness, shock or the cumulative fears of having to meet stressors for which one feels inadequately trained or prepared. This could be coping with a job which is beyond one's capabilities. Having to impart one's skills to others by lecturing or demonstrating when one is shy and tongue tied with students, groups of fellow workers or trainees.

Fear of failure Many jobs have grown and diversified so much in the last few years that one can find oneself placed in situations unsought and consequently become terrified of failure. In addition, with the escalating costs of keeping a home and family going (and often keeping two families going today), the home, which should be a haven where all tensions melt and disappear, is often itself the focus of anxiety in its family members. This is dangerous for health but is perhaps understandable in a country undergoing economic recession, where inflation plays havoc with budgets and where people are strained but dare not give up their jobs in the face of three million unemployed. It is not surprising that we have the biggest bill for tranquillisers this country has ever seen.

Handling anxiety

We have to do three things. First, tackle the problems. Second, tackle the symptoms of high tension, blood pressure and the physical ills the problems have caused. Third, we have to tackle the social side and develop support

184

systems if these are missing in the home. So the remedies are in three different spheres: the intellectual problem solving sphere, the physical sphere and the social sphere. We will deal with these in that order and develop a formula for the first sphere of problem solving.

We have to begin to use the signal of anxiety for what it really is – a signal that something is upsetting our emotional balance. There is probably more than one problem or situation which is undermining our emotional health. Stop, sit down today with pen and paper and write down all the things which you find stressful. Bring these out into the open, from your emotional centres to your thinking areas in the brain. This is where the problems can be solved.

The intellectual sphere

Below are some situations which people find very stressful and how they react to them. They are verbatim, just as received, and the very staccato fashion in which they are reported often masks a great deal of anxiety.

Situation	Emotion
1 Being late for work and appointments.	Anger
2 Getting overdrawn at the bank.	Worry
3 Feeling alone at times. (A successful top executive – married)	Fear
4 Leaving children very early in the morning when they are pleading 'don't go'. (A father – one parent family)	Worry
5 Colleagues getting ahead of me.	Panic, worry and loss of self-esteem
6 Too many things to do.	Frustration and worry
7 Work partners having different objectives.	Depression and negative handling
8 People putting their burdens and problems on me until I can't take any more. (Personnel Officer)	Anger and tears
9 People not understanding what I'm trying to do.	Anger and frustration
10 Living with a partner about to be divorced. (A working mother having taken in son pending his divorce)	Insecurity

185

Situation	Emotion
11 Widowed – money – coping financially.	Worry
12 Working – housekeeping, etc. (A working mother with two children, divorced)	Tired
13 Over drinking, over smoking, over crowded in noisy flat. (Mother working in top job, two children, divorced)	Anger, frustration and worry
14 Telephones constantly ringing. I can't get on with my own very high pile of work. (Secretary in advertising)	Anger, frustration, and finally depression
15 Children waking during the night. (Mother – one-parent family, two children under 5)	Lose temper, hate myself for being unfeeling due to tiredness
16 Visits from superiors.	Panic. No reason, just terrified
17 Pressures at home due to long hours worked.	Guilt, frustration and rows
18 Conflict in personal life over involvement with job.	Withdrawal from partner and resentment
19 Personal relationship with girl friends/friends.	Worry
20 Coping with an invalid mother who suffers from depression.	Anger, worry or depression

When we look at other people's top stressors in this way we feel like saying, 'Well, why doesn't he/she do so and so?' It is easy when you are not in the emotionally confusing situation alternating between the, 'If only life were different,' or 'I'll walk out, then they'll miss me.' When we take the problems out of the emotional level and write them down and present them to our intellectual levels as a problem to be solved the whole thing becomes possible. More than this – it positively can be done.

Write down your most stressful situations

So now to your problems. Write down the situations, things or events which make you most stressed. What is your reaction to them? Think how you really feel about each one. Which emotion predominates? Is it fear, anger, hate or frustration or do you withdraw and run away from

186

it? In order to solve the problems at the thinking level you have to analyse the feeling and recognise it. Only then can you do something about it.

Now look at your problems dispassionately. What are they due to? How many of them could you reduce right away by asserting yourself? Many of our problems are due to not asserting ourselves. No, you do not want a puppy (think of the training, feeding etc, and you *know* that the children will not look after it all the time). No, you do not want your parents, in-laws, children, to stay next weekend, you are too busy. No, you do not want an energetic holiday, you want to lie in the sun and do absolutely nothing. Be quite definite about what to say no to. It is far less exhausting and anxiety-making than 'perhaps' or 'we'll see'.

    No, you cannot socialise until you have got through the outstanding volume of work. (Look at this again – are you absolutely sure that not even one of the bits of work could be done by someone other than you?)

Learn to say 'no'

We can cut out many of our problems by delegating. There are really only a few things which no one else but you can do. Take the home for instance. Everyone can make coffee, tea, toast (even five year-olds with a pop-up toaster), give themselves a bowl of cereal and pour a glass of orange juice. That is breakfast out of the way. Eight year-old children can take care of their own bedrooms. Beds may not be made as you would make them but does it matter? And tidying can be done at the weekend.

    High standards are important and can be maintained if one has the help to do it. When one is head cook, bottle washer, housekeeper, mother and at the same time holding down a 9 to 5 job, then your health and strength are more important to your family than your standards. So delegate happily and close your eyes, but keep just a minimum of standards, and insist on these. It might be no milk bottles on the table or no plastic beakers, but standards, even little ones, are important. Go through your list systematically. Identify the stressor, identify the emotion and then set out to meet that stressor head on and vanquish it.

Delegate and close your eyes

Now that you have identified things or events which make you anxious, tense and stressed, and you have identified the resulting emotion, you have carried out part one of a formula in this intellectual problem-solving technique

Identification

187

which will work for you whatever your stressors: identification. You have identified the stressor and how it affects you. Now you have to imagine that you are an actor or actress learning and immersing yourself in a part until you are word and action perfect in order to develop the techniques which will overcome your particular stressor, whether it is talking to a group, asking for a rise or bringing up a delicate issue with your partner. No matter what it is this will stress proof you.

Perfect preparation

The first essential in this is perfect preparation. Prepare to meet and deal with that stressor head on. Whatever you are funking, dreading or are just plain angry at, prepare to attack it positively. For example, let us take the first of the stressful situations on page 185, the anger, frustration, and for many the fear of being late for appointments, meetings and work and the failure to deliver work on time. This is a prime fear of many people as they feel that so many things are out of their own control. Buses arrive in convoys, trains can be cancelled or arrive late, taxis go by without stopping although empty and time pressures are impossible. This is absolutely true because many of us have an unrealistic view of time today.

We fill up our diaries allowing insufficient time for interviews, for travelling (half hour to get across London when it can take an hour). There are things for which we allow no time at all, for example, telephone calls, both making and receiving, shopping (done on the way to or from work or at lunchtime), washing (thrown into the machine on the way through the kitchen) and preparation time for papers, reports and budgets. Part of perfect preparation to meet these stressors is realistic planning in the diary, allowing time for the eventualities which always happen if you are not prepared for them.

Thorough rehearsal

Part of every actor's life is thorough rehearsal. Whether the stressor you have planned to meet is making that important telephone call, or that suggestion to management which could make your life much easier, or the talk to that group of trainees, rehearse it in your mind until you are absolutely word and action perfect. Then rehearse it until you feel easy and natural and it is a part of you. Just like acting a part, you have to make it convincing.

Confidence

This comes from the earlier parts. Once you have identified, planned and rehearsed in detail to meet your stressor, whatever it may be, you will feel the confidence of the perfectly prepared.

This then is the full formula for the first part of our stress proofing programme.

The programme

1 Identification of the stressor and the emotion it raises in you.
2 Perfect preparation to meet it.
3 Thorough rehearsal of words and action you will take to confront it.
4 Confidence of the fully prepared.

Now the second part is the physical. Look back at the pattern of anxiety on page 185 and you will see that as well as the intellectual sphere it has a physical sphere and a social sphere. All of these have to be tackled.

It is just as vital to deal with the physical as with the intellectual. Anxiety is really stress. Some people have tried to class them as different entities because of different approaches. The physiological changes in the heart, circulation and biochemistry have been the province of the medical world, the psychiatrists and the pathologists, and there the name 'stress' was coined.

The physical sphere

'Anxiety', meanwhile, has been the province of the psychologists. It is, as Professor Scrignar, Clinical Professor of Psychiatry at Tulane University School of Medicine, USA, says, 'Like the proverbial blind man of Indostan touching various parts of an elephant. Clinicians and researchers alike have been studying the same elephant but drawing different conclusions when touching the trunk and then the tail. The response of the central nervous system, autonomic nervous system, endocrine system and end organs are identical whether labelled anxiety or stress.'

So what we are really talking about is 'stress' with all of its symptoms. In anxiety, the underlying emotion which alerts the stress response to switch on and help is often fear. Whether fear of failure, of losing one's love or one's job, the main symptoms may be those of the lungs, heart and circulation, of tightness in the chest, a fast beating heart or difficulties in breathing. They may, on the other hand, be mainly gastro-intestinal – difficulties in swallowing (feeling

'Anxiety' is 'stress'

189

one has a lump in the throat), feeling nauseous or having frequent bowel movements. You need to get the high tension and arousal levels down as well as tackling the problems. To do this turn to Chapter 8 and carry out the First Aid techniques to get you through your day.

Learn to tranquillise

If you are prone to anxiety it would also be helpful to learn to tranquillise yourself because this brings about a rapid lowering of anxiety and it is simple to do. There is nothing mystical or difficult about this simple procedure.

Here is what you do:

1 Choose a room you like and in which you feel at peace. The atmosphere should be conducive to relaxation and comfortably warm. Close the door and make sure you are undisturbed for half an hour.
2 Loosen all tight clothing, take off your shoes and pick a comfortable chair in which you can lie back and feel at peace.
3 Use the calming breathing technique in Chapter 8 to calm and steady you at the start. Close your eyes, lie back and let go. Just be pleased to be at peace and quiet.
4 Pick a word which makes you *feel* peaceful. I use the word 'Peace'. Murmur it softly to yourself then just let it reach and calm the emotional centres of the brain (in the middle). Be aware of the word all the time and of what it means to you. *Feel* peaceful and utterly at rest.
5 Do not worry if your thoughts drift. Just keep the word peace in your mind and let it happen. You are just letting the world go by you for half an hour, and bringing all those tension levels back to normal. At the end of half an hour, come to slowly and take a deep, energising breath. You are rested, calm and tranquil.

Try to keep to the same time every day to do this and the system will gradually become fully relaxed and at peace.

The social sphere

Anxieties, problems and worries tend to get out of hand unless we can keep them in perspective and we can only get this perspective from other people. Friends who will listen to us and reassure us are vitally important to our emotional health. We should be able to rely upon our family for a firm foundation of support, but in addition to this we need one

190

or two very close friends upon whom we can rely and with whom we can really be ourselves, 'warts and all'. Then we need a very wide band of friends of all ages. The different age groups have a different perspective on problems which can be both refreshing and helpful. An ideal situation would be one in which such a group could meet together weekly or fortnightly over a cup of coffee to discuss their own problems and find solutions. The Stress Foundation can help with suggestions in setting up such a group approach. They will suggest topics to discuss and provide useful back-up information in order that you can arrive at solutions of how to handle the problems in your lives.

With these three approaches – the intellectual one of solving the problems with its formula for success, the physical approach, a combination of the techniques in Chapter 8 and of tranquillising, and finally with a ready made support group – you know that you can come through anxiety with your flag of confidence flying high.

CHAPTER 15

Getting the social balance right: develop confidence. Pamper yourself

You are individual and unique. There is no one else in the world like you, not even your identical twin. You have tremendous potential. We all have. Yet we do not use one tenth of this potential, not in personality, charm, poise, brain power, nor in our ability to delight and interest others. Some of us develop poise and balance (models), some of us develop our brain power (academics), and some of us develop our ability to talk and sway others by argument (politicians).

You have tremendous potential

But we all have the potential in our genes at birth to do all of these things. Some of us, it is true, have a greater ability than others for developing a particular part of it. Some have had their potential developed in a particular field through family interest or from good tutors. But luckily it is never too late to develop all sides of our personalities. You must have felt yourself to be different with different people. Some people draw out the happy laughing side of you, others the more serious, and some the more daring side when you 'let your hair down' or 'freak out'. So, as you have discovered, you have many different sides to yourself. What happens though if they are not drawn out? Do you just bury parts of yourself leaving them dormant?

To be really stress proofed

To be really stress proofed we need to be whole and well balanced. So take out all those dormant or buried parts of yourself which you would like to develop, shine them up and surprise those who have only seen one side of you so far.

It is sometimes difficult to develop the sparkling, vivacious sides of ourselves if we have very strong personalities in the family. It is so much easier to sit back and let them hog the limelight. Then, when they have left home, the

192

sitting back quietly has become so habitual that we do not break out unless others drag it out of us. But it is there. If you have been overshadowed by a dominant partner, it is probably difficult for you to know exactly what your potential is. So let us embark on a voyage of discovery and find out what you are really like.

Why not take a little time now to find out? List what you are, what you like and all of your favourite things, the things *you* really like. Not your family, nor your friends. You.

How do I see myself?

Look in a long mirror. How do you stand? Do you have an upright commanding stance? Do you appear confident with head up, ready and willing to meet the world face to face? How do you dress? Would people meeting you think of you as conventional, daring, individualistic, sloppy or modern? What are the colours of your off duty clothes – earthy, conventional, daring, dramatic or folksy?

What do you look like to others?

What is your favourite aftershave, body lotion or perfume? Do you go for the woody scents, the deep musky, male smells, the more feminine light flower fragrances, or the sharper sophisticated notes, which can suit either sex? Think of these in relation to that side of your personality you most want to project to others.

Think, have I very catholic tastes and like most things depending on mood, or have I particular kinds of music which lift my mood if feeling down? How do I feel about classical music? Do I really like opera? Which are my favourites? Jazzy, traditional or modern? Pop – the now almost traditional 60s? Modern – which groups? Folk – which singers?

What is your favourite music?

Now extend this process to considering the rest of your preferences. What are my favourite films, plays, television and radio programmes?
Who are my favourite authors?
When did I last have time to read a book and enjoy it?
What is my favourite food?
How do I really like my eggs done?
What is my favourite sport or game?
When did I last play?

In this way, build up a complete profile of yourself with all of your likes and you could add your dislikes at the same time. The main thing is to begin to think about yourself as an individual quite apart from everyone else; a personality in your own right. Are you really using the things you like to bring you pleasure every day?

You have many qualities. We tend to overlook these when we are highly pressed or a little down and remember only our failures and difficulties. Think now of the good things.

How do other people see you? Give the chart to a friend of the same sex, and then to one of the opposite sex, and ask them to tick the boxes as honestly as they can.

Never Rarely Sometimes Usually Always

Friendly
Sympathetic
Fun to be with
Decisive
Bossy
Witty and amusing
Reliable
Honest
A good listener
A good talker
Stimulating
Generous
Patient
A loyal friend
Exciting to be with
Lively
Intelligent
A good sport
Practical
Understanding
Sexy
Affectionate
Calm
Supportive
Non-jealous
Outgoing
Shy
Imaginative
Full of courage

Look at the list. Be pleased with those qualities which are highly praised. Now what about those hidden assets of yours which do not come across? Dig those out and shine them up and you will be even more popular.

People who are consistently socially competent (as the researchers call popularity) and make friends easily have the following attributes in common:

What makes for popularity?

- They genuinely like people and find them interesting.
- They are good listeners.
- They are able to talk to all kinds of people about many different things.
- They try to set other people at their ease.
- They are direct and decisive (without being blunt); people 'know where they are' with them.
- They are easy to get along with and not moody.
- They are not over critical, but accept people as they are, 'warts and all'.
- They are interested in what people do and so tend to ask many questions.
- The most important factor here for 'social competence' is being genuinely interested in other people; in what they do, in what they think, in their ideas about life. This leads naturally to setting people at their ease and it leads conversation on.

The most popular person I know is a woman who welcomes people in with a 'How lovely to see you.' (emphasised and meant.) 'Do come in. I'm dying to hear how you got on about [or with] so and so, and you're not going until you've told me all about it.' She then settles you on the sofa with many cushions, gets out the drinks and settles back herself expectantly. You know that she is genuinely interested in you and that you have made her day or evening by dropping in.

The most popular person I know

So now you have something to build upon. Your own profile, yourself as others see you, and the qualities which make for easy friendship. So next, would you like to be more poised and make a commanding entry wherever you go? It does wonders for your self esteem and confidence.

195

Develop a commanding carriage

Get the spine into alignment easily and gracefully and without strain.

1 Have two large books ready to hand. These are to raise the head and neck to an easy relaxed level.
2 Have two firm pillows to hand. These are to put under your knees.
3 Lie down on the floor with the head comfortably supported on the books and the legs raised either over the two pillows or, if you can, bring your knees up until your feet are comfortably flat on the floor. This allows the whole of the spine to uncurl and the small of the back to straighten out flat on the floor.
4 Feel your spine lengthening from your neck to your coccyx (your 'tail'). Become aware (do not strain at it) that the whole of your spine is lying easily, flat on the floor and becoming longer naturally.
5 Now feel the whole of the back widening (you have done this in Chapter 8) from the centre of the spine out to the sides.
6 Feel the shoulders widen out and move them out easily to accommodate this. Lay them flat and, feeling 'wide' on the floor, rest the hands lightly on the diaphragm as you do for diaphragmatic breathing.
7 Breathe easily, using the gentle calming breathing which you learned in Chapter 8.
8 'Feel' this widened, lengthened and straightened spine. Recognise the different 'feel' from that which you customarily use. Now aim for this feel all the time, wherever you move.

Poise the head

Set the head easily and gracefully erect.

1 Walk the newly straightened spine over to the nearest wall and have a long mirror facing you.
2 Back up to the wall, let the heels touch the wall, lengthen and widen the spine up against it. Do not strain and get the 'feel' you achieved on the floor.
3 Now release the neck, let your head find its way to the wall naturally. Do not strain any part of you.
4 Rest the back of the head against the wall, letting it join the lengthened, widened spine.
5 Look straight ahead at the mirror, the head should be set easily on the top of the spine. Feel as if a cord is coming from the top, pulling it up easily.

196

6 Make sure that there is no strain. The feeling should be one of release as the small bones of the spine are released from their compressed state and the head is poised. You realise now how far forward the head is sometimes carried and why models look so poised and in command of the situation. They are a head taller.

Keeping this position, move forward gracefully, smoothly and easily, letting the hip movement carry you forward. Forget the 'chin up and tummy in' business. When the spine and head are in a natural alignment everything else goes back naturally to its proper place. You immediately feel more poised, don't you? Do not worry if the alignment is not quite right yet, it will come. You can make quite an entry having gone this far. In your work, the appearance of confidence and of being in command of every situation, does get you noticed, and you are categorised, like it or not, as 'officer' or 'executive' material.

Now that you feel ten feet tall it will not be easy for people to walk all over you. Human nature is odd in a way. Even if people do not mean to be dominating it seems to be 'natural' to take the lead over others who appear to be more self effacing. There must be give and take in all our relationships; with our children (they must learn to be independent too) and with our partners. It is not really fair to one's partner to be dominant all of the time. All of us need care, love and tenderness and sometimes when we feel low we need to be cradled again like a child. At other times it is great to assert oneself and to run the whole gamut of human emotions. Do not get stuck in one mode. So when you feel the need to assert yourself here is how to do it.

Now that you feel great: be great

What is ego strength? It is quite simply strength of your own personality. Part of developing ego strength is what we were doing at the start of this chapter. That is, building up a profile of you, your likes and your dislikes. This is all part of being a person with ego strength. It is also being independent, having a mind of your own and the ability to make your own decisions. It is also about being decisive. Being quite definite about the standards of work you need from others, being definite about the kind of help you need from your partner and from the family. Being quite definite about your own needs and priorities for leading a

Developing ego strength

happy and fulfilled life.

This is why it is important to know what makes us happy.

Now, the following situations are common to many women, but the principle of being quite specific about what you want, and how you act, is equally applicable to us all, male and female alike.

What do you do?

1 You are at the hairdresser's. You asked for the latest hairstyle. It has been done and you look awful. It just does not suit you at all – what do you do?

(a) Just die inside and race home to alter it.

(b) Think, 'Well I might get used to it.'

(c) Say 'Oh Lord, that was a mistake wasn't it, what can we do to alter it?'

2 You have an important report to do by Monday morning. You have set aside Saturday and Sunday to do it. Then you find that your beloved has asked friends down for the weekend. What do you do?

(a) Flare up and have a row.

(b) Think, 'Why does life never go right,' and work all Friday night.

(c) Say, 'Sorry, I should have checked, but I can't possibly entertain this weekend.'

3 You are invited to a party. At 8 pm your partner still hasn't arrived home. What do you do?

(a) Ring the office and ask what has happened.

(b) Ring your friends and say you cannot make it.

(c) Go, and leave a note for your partner to come on and join you.

4 You have a full-time job, two small children and a fair sized house to manage. Your husband always gets home at 7pm, pours a drink and relaxes in front of the television for the evening. What do you do?

(a) Murmur, 'It's all right for some people,' and smoulder and get more and more irritable.

(b) Feel hard done by and get more and more martyred and depressed.

(c) Say something quite specific like, 'Darling will you see the children to bed and read them a story while I prepare food, then we can sit and have a drink before dinner.'

Your reactions

If your answers were mainly (a)s you need action when fed up or hard pressed because you tend to get aggressive or over react. Very many of us who are by nature gentle and

198

unassuming find it difficult to be strong unless we are angry. This is not the way to ego strength. In fact, it is just the reverse. We become frustrated and irritable and add to our tension and arousal levels.

If your answers were mainly (b)s you tend to give in. 'Anything for a quiet life' might well be your motto. But it does not become quiet because people walk all over you. Probably quite unintentionally, but it happens. You could get very depressed unless you become more definite about your own needs.

If your answers were mainly (c)s, great. Yes, you have ego strength. Make them all (c)s now. At the same time, recognise that every other family member has their own needs and priorities and should be decisive about these. There needs to be full and frank discussion and often a compromise will have to be reached. But this is democracy at its best.

Standing and walking in a poised fashion and entering shops or your place of work, slowly and decisively, gives the appearance of a strong personality. Look as if you expect to be noticed and treated as a VIP. Get used to expecting this and never let yourself be elbowed aside by pushy queue jumpers. A ploy of a friend of mine which always works is to say calmly and nicely to anyone thrusting in, 'Oh, well do go ahead if you have an urgent problem.' The thruster apologises and steps back not wanting to be seen as having a problem.
Ego strength in shops

At work, one meets all types of personalities. Some colleagues can be abrasive and outspoken and do not realise how rude they sound to those of a gentler disposition. Decisiveness here is to say quite quietly and calmly that you are not used to being spoken to so rudely and that you find it quite distressing. This will help the other to modify the offensive behaviour and so improve his/her relationships. So it is doing them a good turn to act and not withdraw or leave. Bosses can be inconsiderate, being more aware of the work they want to get out, than of how overloaded their PA is on a Friday night. If you get a great deal of work and you know there is no hope of finishing it all before you go home, ask which is the most urgent because you have only the time to do a certain amount and state that amount.
Ego strength at work

As you can see, being decisive helps everyone to know

199

exactly how they stand which allows them to make decisions in their turn. It is therefore helpful social behaviour. What is not helpful is keeping silent and then getting uptight, moody or even aggressive, banging doors, going and getting drunk or having a quiet cry. People do not know why you are uptight unless you tell them. It is far better to avoid such a situation by not having a reason to get edgy.

So, to develop ego strength:

1 Practise the standing and walking tall.
2 Practise the 'expectation' of being noticed wherever you go.
3 Perfect your technique with queue jumpers, nicely and quietly.
4 Know what your priorities are from your profile of yourself.
5 Decide upon one or two things which will make your life easier at home, particularly if you are a one-parent family. Make the children get breakfast, ask the eldest to shop and put the young children to bed or wash up if you cook, or vice versa.
6 Do not wait until you feel stressed and fatigued because you will not be able to be unemotional in discussion. Decide upon what you need and state it easily and calmly. The family is a team and each one feels more involved if they have their own responsibilities.
7 Be prepared to discuss and compromise so that everyone can have priorities respected in their turn.

Love and pamper yourself

Mainly (though not exclusively) for women

A large part of developing an outstanding personality is to love yourself. Unless you like yourself as a person, feel at ease with yourself and know that you have something to offer to others you will never feel easy in friendship or in love.

So here, briefly, is how to start a love affair with yourself.

When we lead very full lives we do not have the time to pamper ourselves as we did when we had only ourselves to consider. Take a morning or afternoon and set aside four hours for pampering.

You will need:

200

1 A really warm bathroom.
2 A loofah, nailbrush, bath soap and bath oil and a pumice stone for your bath.
3 A large warm towel to wrap up in afterwards.
4 Shampoo for hair and a conditioner.
5 A bottle of body lotion.
6 Nail scissors, file, orange sticks, cotton wool, and a buffer for your nails.

Now take plenty of time to luxuriate in the bath using a well-soaped loofah to rub off all the dead cells. You may find you will need the pumice stone for your heels. Lie back in the bath, soak in the warmth and the perfume from your bath oil and relax. Practise the feel of the lengthened and widened spine again and breathe away gently and calmly, loving every minute of it.

Now climb out slowly, wrap yourself in your warm towel and when dry take your bottle of body lotion and massage your whole body from the throat and neck down to your toes. You do not have to learn a special technique for this to be effective, just firm stroking of the skin all over will complete the relaxation started in the bath and allow all of the muscles to relax and lengthen instead of being short, tense and knotted up. Pay particular attention to the back of the neck as this is often tense. Work from the shoulders up and from the centre of the neck out with the three middle fingers of each hand.

Slap off the fat

The thighs, if fatter than you would like, can take slapping rhythmically, or kneading (just like kneading dough). This helps the breaking down of the fat cells. Avoid any red threads of veins or varicose veins if doing this on the legs. Finish by massaging the feet (the whole of the soles which usually get little attention) and pay particular attention to your toes which are usually cramped into shoes. Pull each toe gently up and out, lengthening it, and massage all around each one.

A new hairstyle?

Lie down, relax for half an hour after your massage, luxuriating in the tingling feel of this just as you did in the warmth of the bath. Then do your hair and nails. After your hair shampoo and conditioner, how about trying out a new way of doing your hair? Experiment. Comb it in different ways, perhaps all forwards from the crown if you have always combed it to one side or the back. What about

201

trying a tint? There are now plenty on the market that will wash out if you do not like the result. This could be the start of a new you. Keep up this pampering routine at least once a week. It will pay dividends for your confidence and you will never be caught out ungroomed.

Developing friendships

Now that you have developed a strong ego and have become more confident and self-assured through this, how do you go about making friends? It is very simple, really. There are three stages:

1 Developing a nodding acquaintanceship.
2 Developing a talking acquaintanceship.
3 Working at developing friendship.

Developing a nodding acquaintance-ship

First of all you have to go where people are. You cannot develop a nodding acquaintanceship with anyone if you travel in your closed car to your closed office and travel back the same way to your flat. Go by public transport, catch the same bus, train or coach and you are bound to see the same people every day doing the same thing. Smile at first, then nod and say, 'Good morning', and soon you will be at the 'weather stage'. This will soon develop to a talking acquaintanceship if you are friendly and show that you are pleased to see the person again.

Proximity

There is a now famous piece of research which was carried out to discover how people developed friendships.* There happened to be new college residences ready for an intake of new students, all strangers to one another. This was felt to be too good an opportunity to miss for the psychologists at the college. Now, the buildings were U-shaped, and it was found that those with most friends were those in the busiest passing areas. Those at the two ends of the U had less than half the number of friends than everyone else. So friendship has little to do with shyness or personality. It has everything to do with just being where people are and seeing them every day.

* This research was done by Festinger et al in the USA (Festinger L, Schechter S and Back K, *Social Pressures in Informal Groups: A Study of a Housing Community*, New York, Harper & Row, 1950).

Studies since then among medical students and college students have remarked on the same things. It is usual to seat people by the first letter of their surname and friendships develop. It is quite amazing how many As marry As. This is just because they sit together day after day. So getting beside people every day is the first requisite. Smiling when you notice them is the next. The final stage is talking to them to discover if you have likes in common. If you have, then you are well on the way to friendship.

'A's marry 'A's

People like people who like them. We all feel flattered if we know people like us or think well of us even if we are not too keen on them. But research shows that when people perceive that they are liked by someone they tend to like that person in return.

Will they like you?

People also like others who have similar tastes to their own, so make sure that you talk about the things you like and also those you dislike. These can be the start of friendships. Very close friendships take a long time to develop usually; they have to be worked at and they have to be maintained. This takes time and energy and is very difficult if you have the kind of job which takes all of your time and all of your energy.

Ideally, it is a good idea to keep in your diary at the end of the week – your social time – names of your friends with their telephone numbers with whom you have not been in contact recently. Ring them up. If you do not, it is amazing how time can pass without renewing contact, particularly if they or you have moved away. Also, keep a stock of stamped cards and write one or two on your way to and from work.

Plan in your diary

At the same time you must develop a group of friends near at hand with whom you feel at ease. Meet these frequently even if it is only for a coffee and a short get together. Friends are your support group, essential to a stress proofed system and essential to your health. If you do not have friends dropping in to see you there is something wrong. Look very carefully at your welcoming techniques. Are you always pleased to see them and do you make them welcome and show that you are interested in them? Or do you immediately launch into your own problems and talk about the terrible day you have had and all your other problems and difficulties? If everyone has stopped dropping in, you will have to work very hard on getting your friendships developed again.

If you have moved

It is very hard to move to a new area some distance from highly supportive friends. When this happens the only thing to do is to invite them down for a day or a weekend. Old, trusted friends who know you well are worth their weight in gold and they need treasuring.

Becoming and staying a good lover
We have noted before that the sex urge goes when we are stressed. The system is not able to carry out all its normal functions when it is at a very low ebb through depression, frustration or boredom, nor at the other end of the scale when we are going full pelt and using up all our energies in our work. If you are in this situation, it should now be remedied. Getting back to being a good lover after having been stressed takes a little working at.

Being empathic to need

Take time to look at your lover, whoever he or she is, tell them when they look nice, notice when they have had a haircut, or are wearing something new or different and show that you appreciate this. It will develop the wish to look nice for you. Be perceptive to their mood. After a heavy day of non-stop talk the one need is for blessed silence; if one has been all day working alone the need is to talk. Often one gets a situation where one partner needs silence and the other to talk. In this case, leaving the one with a drink and quiet while the other goes round to see a friend for an hour will enable them to talk together easily over a late meal and enjoy it.

Love and affection

Love is a basic human need, as vital as food and shelter. Babies need cuddling, children need hugging and kissing, adolescents need cuddling, particularly when upset or down and when things have gone wrong. Adults in the family need hugging and the closeness of touch. Your friends need the friendliness of touch, the hand on the arm and a hug when arriving. Unfortunately, in our society many people have not had this basic need met, perhaps because their parents had personality problems and were unable to show normal natural affection. The result is that as adults in their turn they feel uncomfortable about hugging and caressing their children, believing it to be sexual.

204

The truth is that cuddling, hugging, stroking and caressing is a basic need which goes throughout the animal kingdom, particularly in those species which like us humans are gregarious and live in groups. Research has shown that infant monkeys brought up without cuddling and clinging are not normal in behaviour. The absence of cuddling leads to aggressive behaviour, timidity, frigidity and non-normal behaviour as an adult; difficulty in courtship practices, in mating and in mothering. Cuddling makes behaviour gentle. Research into humans has also shown the need for touching and caressing. Even stroking and caressing a small animal can relieve stress and tension. The elderly lonely, the handicapped and 'difficult' children all become much better when they have a small pet to stroke and caress.

Caressing is 'gentling'

With this basic human need in mind, caressing, cuddling, stroking and the closeness of touch is as essential in marriage or lovemaking as the sexual act itself. In fact, it is much more important because without it the act itself is stripped of a great deal of its sexuality of feeling.

Caressing and lovemaking

Bring back the sensuality to life. Anything which enhances the feel of things through the skin will heighten sensuality, heighten the feel of air, of sun, of silk or fur on your bare skin. After a warm bath together, turn the lights down low in the bedroom, throw a fur rug over the bed lie face down and massage each other's backs in turn. Take in the entire back from the neck and shoulders down to the feet. Use body lotion to make the feel silky. Make sure that the room is warmer than usual. This in itself heightens sensuality. This treatment will bring the circulation to the skin and you will both feel great. You may feel much more sexually alive at the end but this is not the point of the exercise. Cuddling and caressing afterwards and lying in each other's arms to sleep will take all the tensions and worries of the day away and lead to high stress proofing for both of you.

Developing sensuality

PART III

Stress-induced illnesses and professional help

The first part of this book helped you with the identification of stress in all its forms, and Part II explained in detail how to deal with it. However, some people, and perhaps this includes you, will have read this book a little late, and perhaps you are already suffering from an illness or a distressing symptom which your doctor tells you is due to stress. While the problem has been identified, there seems to be little help available to you. Nonetheless, you will want to know two things immediately. First, how to get better, and then how to be sure that your illness, whether it is a heart attack, an ulcer or a lump in the throat that makes eating difficult, does not happen again. This third part is written especially for you. Here there are three chapters. Chapter 16 describes the people who can help you in both orthodox and complementary medicine. We use the term 'complementary' because there are therapies and healing techniques that add to and complement our orthodox medicine. They go well together and will do so more and more in the future. In complementary medicine it is important that you only consult well-qualified practitioners and this chapter tries to make sure that you learn how to do this. To this end the chapter lists only those complementary therapies that have a proven record of success in treating the whole person. If you want to explore other possibilities, a fuller list of what is possible is given in Appendix 2. In this chapter we will deal with three different groups of help:

Orthodox medicine	The Family Doctor
	The Psychiatrist
Orthodox psychology	The Psychotherapist
	The Psychologist
Complementary medicine	Acupuncture
	Herbalism
	Homeopathy
	Naturopathy
	Chiropractic
	Osteopathy
	Counselling

So, first we will deal with the orthodox treatment for stress, and look at the roles of the family doctor and the psychiatrist, their training and the help that they will be able to give. Orthodox medicine, as taught in all the medical schools in Great Britain, is unquestionably the best in the world. Therefore, it follows that if your stressors have already triggered off a known disease or illness, your own doctor is the best person to diagnose and treat it, or to refer you to the best consultant if a specialist is needed. Only when you have been through this process and discovered that, luckily, organic damage has not yet resulted from your stressors, should you consider complementary medicine. There are several good reasons for tackling your problem in this order, but a major one is the interpretation of your subjective experience of pain. There have been known cases where a heart condition has been treated as 'indigestion due to stress' (both can produce 'pain across the chest'). A general practitioner would have been alerted and have immediately taken blood pressure and an EEG. So I would advise strongly that your first visit must be to your own family doctor, but go to him thinking of your visit as the first stage in a process of discovery. Give your doctor a full and accurate description of what you feel, when and for how long you have experienced it, so that he may interpret these signs and symptoms and match them against known possible conditions. The discovery of what is wrong is the crucial starting point, and once the condition has been diagnosed, the treatment may be to assist your own immunity and defence systems to combat and overcome the invaders if pathogenic organisms have been found, to remove a badly infected part by surgery to allow an organ to function properly again, or perhaps to help your tissue repair system if tissues have suffered badly.

Chapter 17 deals with the part that the stresses and strains of life play in all this and the type of illnesses that they are most likely to trigger off. The illnesses and conditions are listed alphabetically for ease of reference. First, the recognised illnesses and then some distressing symptoms. Suggestions are given for the relief of these conditions and for their prevention in the future once they have been cured – always from the point of view of their stress content. For this reason we include a note on cancer because of the fear which this condition causes. It is currently held in the same dread as was 'the white death' (Tuberculosis) only a century ago, and we do have to remember, understand and believe that, like Tuberculosis, cancer is curable in its early stages. It is the recognition of the condition which should concern us, not the fear of its final stages, because it should never be allowed to get that far.

So the problem of cancer is dealt with purely from the viewpoint of it's prevention and it's early recognition. For these reasons, we do not go into the details of the different types of the disease, their probable causes and their treatment. What we do is to find out what people know about it, what the difference in belief is between those who do go for check ups and those who don't. One of the basic reasons would seem to be fear.

It may help you to be less afraid of cancer if you can understand that the cells are very like our own body cells which divide and multiply to make more tissue for us. Some cells (cancer cells) appear to rebel and go their own way and our own defence system usually engulfs them and gets rid of them as unwanted by the system because they have become alien. Alien cells are immediately treated as invaders and killed. So the best way of preventing cancer is to keep our defence and immunity systems up to peak condition. Read the Lifestyle chapter in Part 2 in order to know how to do this most effectively from the physical point of view. Develop your friendships and seek and pursue happiness whenever and wherever you can, because positive emotional health is the very best way of raising the tone and level of function of the whole system.

The early warning signs of cancer are given in Chapter 17, and do take note of these. To be absolutely on the safe side, do go to your doctor with any persistent changes in your normal health ie a change which has lasted for at least

2 weeks and is continuing, whether it be bruises that don't go away, unnatural fatigue combined with loss of appetite, sores on the lips which don't heal etc etc. These may not indicate cancer but they do indicate your normally excellent defence and immunity systems are having difficulty in coping with something and it is as well to find out what and put it right.

Remember that you are not alone in this, it is for this reason that the first chapter in this Part III spells out the help available from sources in addition to your own family doctor.

So the first chapter in this Part is *People who can help us*, and the second is *The stress illnesses*. Then we come to the final chapter which moves outwards from you, widening the emphasis through you to your community. In it we suggest what you, now much more knowledgeable in many aspects of stress, can do to reduce the anxieties of your family, your friends and all those with whom you come into close contact. It is up to all of us today to share our knowledge and so to attempt to improve the quality of life for all. Significant movements can result from very small beginnings. From misery, anxiety and despair can arise (like Phoenix from the ashes) groups of people willing to come together to identify their problems and to offer mutual support and aid. This can be particularly helpful in facing up to and combatting stressors, and Phoenix Groups might be quite a good name, or even Phoenix Stress Foundation Groups as you would certainly have the backing of the Stress Foundation in launching such a venture.

CHAPTER 16

People who can help us

Do we go to our family doctor for help early enough? The answer seems to be no. The majority of the population, and this seems to apply more to men than to women, do not go until they have an incapacitating problem such as difficulty in breathing, pain in the chest, or pain in the stomach (which has become so accustomed to antacid pills that they no longer help). But if we did go, what help could we expect? We should expect, and get, a great deal of help. He is the most qualified person in your community to look after your health, or rather your illnesses. He has had six years of training, encompassing every branch of medicine, surgery and psychiatry. In addition, there is now a compulsory extra three years of training to become a member of the Royal College of General Practitioners. Two of these years are spent in hospital as a Registrar working under a consultant in the various specialisations, and one year out in general practice. Further, he has had access to the best specialists and having worked with many of them, his advice on who to see for a general opinion or specialist treatment, is invaluable.

Your family doctor

He is, in fact, a specialist in general medicine. This is why he is the logical starting point for any symptoms or sign of illness. Nine years of experience, even before becoming your family doctor, is the best available help. If nothing abnormal is found after exhaustive tests for all the possibilities, and the symptoms remain, the news is good in that it is an indication that you have caught your stressors in time before they have done any organic damage. But now comes the crunch, because you want to get better and your family doctor cannot, with the best will in the world, take the time to find out what your stressors are, nor to help you to reduce the tensions and stop the long-term biological reactions that are now playing havoc with your normal functioning. All he can do is to attempt to quieten the

Specialist in general medicine

211

system down with tranquillisers. These will give you a breathing space in which to digest Part II of this book thoroughly and carry out the self-help practices set out there. It is, however, essential that you have been through the discovery process first to be sure that there is nothing organically wrong. You are in time to tackle the stressors before they do you any real harm, and for this you should be very thankful. Admittedly, and ironically, most of us feel much better if our doctor says, 'Yes, you have a gastric ulcer and here is your diet,' rather than, 'There is nothing organically wrong with you so it is probably nervous indigestion brought on by stress,' but logically we should be delighted that our stressors have not yet breached our defences.

Unfortunately, the stress process is complex and multi-disciplinary. You need not only the medical side of endocrinology, pathology and immunology, but also neuro-psychology and counselling skills, so few GPs are able to interpret all this and most are at a loss to know what to do other than to offer us a temporary calming period. However, that is not at all a bad thing. With two weeks of calm we can get Part II under our belts, and tackle our stressors with renewed strength.

The psychiatrist   If by any chance you are still highly anxious, or really feel that you cannot tackle this problem alone, ask your GP if he can refer you to a good psychiatrist. The psychiatrist is a specialist in disorders of thought, feelings and behaviour. In one sense you could say that all illness affects our thoughts, feelings and behaviour, so the psychiatrist is really the nearest approach we have in the Western world to a system of caring for the whole individual. Psychiatrists are doctors who have had a six-year general training and have then spent three or more years specialising in psychological medicine. They could be called the specialists in stress for they deal with anxiety and depression, neuroses and phobias. They also deal with other conditions such as schizophrenia and other psychoses, mental defects and immature personalities. It is probably the latter side of their work that attracts most attention and leads patients to believe that psychiatrists only deal with mental illness. Unfortunately, there are not sufficient psychiatrists to go round and only five per cent of patients who visit their GPs for anxiety or depression ever get referred to a psychiatrist for treatment. You should, nonetheless, feel entirely free

212

to discuss a possible referral with your doctor.

A psychotherapist is well able to deal with stress, particularly when it arises from long-standing problems. These would include those stemming from early childhood or the troubled teens that we have tried unsuccessfully to thrust out of our minds. The psychotherapist aims to bring these conflicts back to the conscious mind in order that they can be solved and settled once and for all. He may be a doctor with special training, but more usually he is a psychologist or holds a degree in the social sciences or the equivalent. His psychotherapy training on top of his qualifications is three or four years, and includes the psychoanalytical theories of Freud and Jung as well as the newer theories. It would include supervised clinical work with patients and a personal analysis to clear up any deep-seated problems. Psychotherapy has been called the talking cure because it is, essentially, the talking through of problems. It is helpful for any deep-seated emotional difficulties and for problems in emotional and social behaviour. It gets at the causes of such conditions and seeks to eliminate them, not just to alter the behaviour itself as does 'behavioural' psychology. *Caution*: It is possible to practise psychotherapy in England without training, so do write to the association listed in Appendix 2.

The psychotherapist

Psychology has recently come to the fore in the treatment of stress. You will remember that the psychiatrist has done an additional three years' training in psychological medicine, after his basic six-year training in medicine. He has studied the brain, its thought processes, its function and what can go wrong. The psychologist on the other hand has had a total of three years' training, studying only the normal person in health, together with his personality, behaviour and what makes him an individual, ie his values, attitudes, prejudices and how they are formed. Any one of these aspects is fascinating in itself, and after training, psychologists tend to concentrate on a single aspect such as behaviour or personality. Many concentrate on the brain with its thought and language, or lean towards the function of the brain itself, and how it in turn affects one's total function. Some of these, specialising in the growth of intelligence and thought, become educational psychologists (Diploma in Education) and then train further, as I did myself, in the workings of the brain itself (neurology) and

The psychologist

213

take a Doctorate (PhD) in neuro-psychology. It is important to look at qualifications, for there are many psychologists who, in an attempt to show their preference for work in a particular field, call themselves 'behavioural', 'cognitive' or 'clinical' (working with patients) which may not indicate further training. Really all psychologists with their basic three-year degree are behavioural and cognitive, and able to complement the work of the GP.

Today, behavioural psychology is heard of more and more in the treatment of stress, and so it needs a full explanation. The present-day guru of the behavioural school of psychology is an American Professor, B F Skinner. The behaviourists say that all behaviour can be shaped, that is to say that you can get the behaviour that you want from animals (even birds) and humans, by rewarding the behaviour you like and want, and punishing the behaviour you do not want. You do not have to worry about the brain and the deep unconscious causes of anti-social behaviour or violence – all you have to do is to shape the behaviour you want. Skinner, in order to demonstrate this, taught pigeons to play ping-pong by painstakingly rewarding each natural action with beak and head, until the full repertoire of behaviour was built up. It is important to emphasise that they were 'normal' birds with no neuroses, psychoses or mental defects.

Today, behavioural psychologists undertake to alter undesirable behaviour such as violence, treat conditions such as agoraphobia (a fear of going out in the open), and seek to alter the behaviour of smokers and alcoholics who want to change their habits. Some are moving into the field of stress and seek to alter the behaviour of the depressed and the anxious. With stress, particularly, it is important to discover the causes, ie the problems that give rise to the depressions and anxieties. It is also vital if one has an endogenous depression, to have this treated with the particular chemical, the shortage of which is giving rise to the complaint. So again, in all cases and for all symptoms, start with the family doctor.

Complementary medicine

The complementary therapies listed here are those that have been found to be most useful for the various illnesses or symptoms associated with stress. They are also included because qualified therapists are available with a recognised training behind them.

The therapies are: Acupuncture
Herbalism
Homeopathy
Naturopathy
and the two manipulative therapies
Chiropractic
Osteopathy

The last two therapies have been found to be most effective for low back pain, painful joints and migraine, all of which are frequently triggered off, or intensified, by stress.

The acupuncturist

His therapies have been used in China for more than 2000 years. The theory is that a network of channels criss-cross the body carrying to organs, tissues and all parts of the body and brain the essential energy supply. These channels are thought to regularise the function of the whole. Illness is thought to be due to malformation or stoppage in these channels. The treatment involves stimulation of the affected channels by pressure or by the insertion of needles. Several kinds of needles are used, but the normal ones are thin and their insertion is often not felt. A number of needles are used and they are left in place for a few minutes. If aggravation or worsening of the symptoms occurs, it is often a sign that your condition can be helped by the treatment. You will usually need at least six sessions in order to feel improvement. Treatment works by mobilising your own self-regenerative and self-healing mechanisms in the body. It has been found helpful for many of the stress disorders such as tension headaches, migraine, sinusitis, asthma, hypertension and stomach or bowel disorders.

The herbalist

In the industrialised West, we almost stopped phytotherapy (treatment by herbs) in the second half of the twentieth century. But it was only a pause. It is now growing strongly again because of the attempt to go back to natural substances and to clear our systems of toxic drugs. The extent of this return can be seen in the statistics for 1974.

In that year* exports of herbs to the industrialised countries were:

* (Source: WHO, 1983, *Traditional Medicine and Health Care Coverage*)

250 tonnes of mint
200 tonnes of verbena
150 tonnes of lime blossom
100 tonnes of camomile
 45 tonnes of eucalyptus leaves
 30 tonnes of orange blossom
 30 tonnes of star anise

The Faculty of Herbal Medicine was started in England in the 1940s and this was followed in 1964 by the formation of the National Association of Medical Herbalists, and these are the two main training centres for herbalists. There is also a Tutorial School of Herbal Medicine in Kent. We have about 12,000 practising herbalists, and herbal remedies are available in over 600 health food stores. Full lists of these are given in the Herb Society's magazine called *The Herbal Review*. The herbalist in this country prepares plants according to the need of his patient using the appropriate mixtures. Our bodies seem to be well adapted to plant cures and we have used them since time immemorial. Animals still seek out plants to eat if they are sick just as our primitive ancestors once did. It is thought that they act by mobilising the body's own regenerative powers and in doing this the right environment is created for natural healing to take place. There are no side effects as there are with drugs, and as the body does not become hooked on herbs, there are no withdrawal symptoms. Their action depends upon what is needed – varying from the robust to the subtle and gentle. With the rise of herbalism in the West, and the consequent over-harvesting of crops, there is concern that some plants of benefit to man are becoming an endangered species. American Ginseng (*Panax quinque folius*), believed to be useful for stress, is one of these. Nothing dramatically curative has been found when Ginseng has been analysed into its constituent parts, but it is possible that this again is a case where the whole is more than the sum of its parts.

The homeopathist

This medical discipline was introduced in 1810 by Samuel Hahnemann, a German doctor. He observed that not all symptoms we have are those of the actual disease. What we see and feel is the reaction of our immune and defence systems in their effort to combat the disease. He decided that a system of medicine based on helping these healing processes would be more effective than the existing cura-

216

tive techniques. In order to overcome a particular illness, the homeopathist has to find a remedy which, when administered to the patient, stimulates the same response as his own defence system. This may well take a long time. The homeopathist therefore needs a great deal of experience in exactly what the homeopathic remedies do in the body. Typically, the training is the six years of medicine plus three years of intensive study in the homeopathic techniques. These are harmless to the system because the amounts used are minute. When the right one is administered, the patient's symptoms immediately become much more pronounced before eventually disappearing with a full return to health. In England, we have five homeopathic hospitals in the National Health Service – London, Glasgow, Liverpool, Bristol and Tunbridge Wells. Nearly 400 doctors practise homeopathy and prescriptions can be had from them either under the National Health Service or privately. Homeopathic remedies are also sold in chemists' shops and health food stores, and from them you can obtain a list of what to take for different illnesses. However, self-diagnosis is always dangerous and it is far better to consult a recognised practitioner. Homeopathy is useful for reversing the trend of diabetes, bronchial asthma, arthritis, skin eruptions and all emotional disorders. So it is invaluable for conditions brought on by stress or made worse by stress or tension.

The naturopathist

This is the oldest and the simplest of the complementary medicines. It is really a philosophy of a natural way of life seeking a pure mind in a healthy body. Perhaps one of the most telling statements about the theories of naturopathy is one by Rudolf Virchow (1821–1902). He said that germs seek their natural habitat which is diseased tissue and that they do not create the diseased tissue. In the same way, mosquitoes seek stagnant water – they do not make the water stagnant. The naturopathist, therefore, is intent on keeping the body, mind and spirit – the total individual – in a natural, healthy state. When he is ill, an attempt at a cure is sought by natural means using:
Water: preferably from natural springs or mineral spas, but if this is not possible, herbs or mineral salts added to bath water.
Air: allowing as much fresh air as possible to get to the body.
Exercise: free movement in the fresh air.

Fresh food: most naturopathists advocate fresh, raw vegetables and fruit with an occasional fast to cleanse the system, and they disallow all unnatural foods such as white flour and refined sugar.

In other words, a great deal of naturopathy is sound common sense. It is saying, in effect, do not overeat rich food, do not drink too much unnatural liquid such as coffee, tea and alcohol, and ensure plenty of fresh air, rest and sleep. If you do this, they say, you will remain healthier longer, and with this every doctor would agree.

The chiropractor

Both chiropractics and osteopathy originated in the USA in the second half of the 19th century. The chiropractor needs a great deal of education and training because he deals with the spine by direct manipulation. It is possible to practise in Britain without training or registration and so it is essential that one contacts the British Chiropractors Association which maintains a register of members, all of whom have graduated from recognised chiropractic colleges. (See Appendix 2.) The complaints most frequently helped are low back pain (lumbago), sciatica and headaches caused by muscle tension in the neck. Occasionally, a malformation of the spine, resulting from the way we stand or use it can cause numb sensations, pain in muscles or pins-and-needles. X-rays will usually reveal the problem, for example, signs of arthritis or 'wear and tear' will show up in the X-ray and the chiropractor will show this to you, explain their significance, and talk over the remedy. If he is not able to help in your particular case he will say so and refer you back to your own family doctor.

The osteopath

The stresses and strains of modern living give rise to tensions in different groups of muscles. The consequence of that is that we hold ourselves differently in order to compensate, and then throw out a shoulder or a hip or some other part of our anatomy. This in turn affects the functioning of inside organs that become displaced. The principle of osteopathy is that 'structure governs function'. When the structure is put out of gear, it affects all other parts of the body which rely upon a balanced skeletal structure. The osteopath puts the structure back together again by manipulation. This sounds similar to the chiropractor. The difference is that osteopaths use more massage techniques as they work with tension in muscle groups and the soft tissues as well as with joints. Perhaps the greatest

218

difference is that osteopaths believe that their main curative effect is on the circulation as a whole, whereas chiropractors believe that they affect the nervous system by the manipulation of the spine because branches of the autonomic nervous system are carried in the spinal column.

There is now, for the first time, a National Register of Counsellors who are able to help you with your problems, whatever they are. Counsellors come from many walks of life. Some have originally qualified in social work, nursing, teaching, sociology or psychology, and have felt the need to work with people in the community. There are those who specialise in children's problems, the problems of those at school and in college, with family problems or with specific problems such as alcoholism. Practically every kind of human problem is dealt with. In order to understand the problems they meet, counsellors listen, after which they use their skills with the client to arrive at workable solutions. They do not psychoanalyse as the psychotherapists or the psychoanalysts do, nor do they attempt, like 'behavioural psychologists', to shape behaviour. They are in essence 'problem oriented' people helping others to solve their own problems in ways which will work for them.

Counsellors

If you need constructive help in coping with your difficulties, the counsellor provides a good complementary back-up to the family doctor who does not have the time to find out what the stresses are which give rise to your symptoms of stress. Some large general practices already employ a counsellor for this purpose one or two days a week, and some counsellors are attached to Health Centres. These will mainly be qualified social workers who have taken a recognised counselling course.

A new and unique association has been formed, by doctors, for doctors who are interested in providing not just orthodox medical care but who want to go further and provide care for the whole individual. This is of great interest for us in the field of stress. Doctors who become members of this association will take full responsibility for the patient's total health and will, when necessary, be prepared to call upon other effective techniques such as acupuncture and osteopathy in addition to more orthodox treatment. Further, there will be an emphasis on self help with the doctor aiming to enlighten the patient about his

Orthodox medicine meets complementary medicine

illness and how he can improve his own health. The doctor and patient will work together more as a partnership in health care rather than continuing the dependent patient-doctor relationship as has so often happened in the past. The association is called the British Holistic Medical Association and it has a list of doctors who are interested in this approach.

CHAPTER 17

The stress illnesses

Should we have any group of illnesses labelled the 'stress illnesses' when, as we have seen already, any long-term interference with our immunity and defence system can result in any illness from the common cold to cancer? Most illnesses, surely, could come into this category? This is absolutely true and so we will restrict the illnesses to those which could be brought about by the long-term effects of the stress chemicals themselves. At the same time, it is important to state that other factors are involved, particularly in the type of illness any individual may have. These factors are heredity, personality, lifestyle and one's weakest link.

Heredity always plays an important part simply because our systems are far more likely to react in the same way as our forefathers' whose genes – the blueprint for our own design – we carry, than in a strange way. Personality and lifestyle we have already covered fully in Chapters 6 and 10. For most of us, the weakest link is the result of previous illness or an accident. It is the part of the body that tires first when we are stressed and fatigued. All of these factors interact. For example, if we have parents who have had heart attacks and we also have a type A, hard-driving, ambitious personality with anger reactions; live a lifestyle in which we take little exercise, eat huge over-rich, highly spiced food with lashings of cream and butter, we had better give it all up and become a village postman without even a bicycle.

If on top of this damaging lifestyle, we are distressed by the various crises which happen to us a stress illness is almost inevitable. The reasons are set out in graph form below. (Only the immunity/illness aspects are given. For example, STH is the growth hormone and has many functions in the body as well as its effect in combatting infection.)

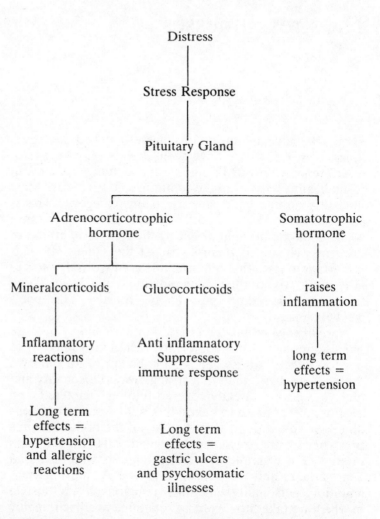

As well as the long-term effects of high inflammatory reactions which result in illness as well as the immuno-suppressive effects of the glucocorticoids, the different groups are, as it were, at odds with each other. In normal health it would not be possible for over-large amounts of these steroids to be in the body at the same time. The effective and delicate feedback systems keep a careful control – except when we are in dire need and cry HELP! Then the stress response pulls out all its big guns to keep us going even at the risk of illness.

So some of the symptoms and illnesses with which we are concerned are:

1 *Allergic reactions*
Allergies and asthma
2 *Digestive difficulties*
Indigestion and dyspepsia, heartburn, gastritis, gastric ulcer, ulcerative colitis, irritable bowel syndrome
3 *Heart conditions*
Hypertension
4 *Skin and joint conditions*
Atopic eczema
Psoriasis
Urticaria
Rheumatoid arthritis
5 *Significant stress component*
Late-onset diabetes
The cancers

Allergic reactions

We hear a great deal about allergies today. We can, it seems, become allergic to anything: to strawberries, milk, chocolate, eggs, cats, birds, flowers, trees and so the eternal list goes on. An American even obtained a divorce because he proved to the satisfaction of the court that he was allergic to his wife. Many of us would say that we are becoming allergic to the 20th century.

An allergy is an abnormal sensitivity of the body to a particular substance and the body reacts by streaming at the eyes or nose, coming out in a rash, wheezing and breathing difficulties, or by pains in the joints. The basic cause is unknown although we do know that over-long action of the mineralcorticoids can cause it (see page 222). In some people there is a disposition to develop allergies which is hereditary. It is as if their immune system lacks a protective substance. For example, a parent can have eczema, one child asthma and another child hay fever. The condition can be triggered by stress. For example, the symptoms might arise just before an examination or, in an adult, after a bereavement. Other emotional traumas can trigger it. The condition itself, particularly eczema in a child and asthma in an adult, can be made much worse by the stress of having it. Allergies are difficult to treat, particularly the multitudinous food allergies, and it is well worthwhile, if you are getting nowhere with orthodox medicine, to try complementary medicine. Herbalists and homeopaths can both be helpful, and if you seem to be allergic to everything, acupuncture may be the answer for you. However, be sure to apply to the qualified practitioners given in Appendix 2.

Asthma

This is an allergic reaction to a variety of substances from pollen to drugs – even aspirin – and to some foodstuffs. In an attack of asthma, the breathing suddenly becomes very laboured and difficult. The bronchial tubes which carry the air in and out of the lungs narrow suddenly through muscular tension in the tubes themselves, and through the sticky mucus which they secrete in their attempt to drive out the allergens causing the attack. When this happens, sit the patient up to give the lungs full expansion, loosen any tight clothing, ring for the doctor at once and reassure the patient (who is terrified his breathing will stop which in turn increases the tension in the chest). The doctor will be able to give immediate help and steroids will bring about a dramatic change in a very few hours. So, calm the patient down and try to get him to breathe gently. The severity and length of an attack depends upon the patient's age, state of health, the number of allergens ingested and his emotional state. In most cases, the asthmatic has a sensitive trigger to stress and reacts quite strongly to many different kinds of stressors which would leave the bulk of the population untouched. For example, a heavy meal, hearty laughter, straining at stool, or a slight set-back can all be powerful stressors and precipitate an attack.

The treatment

The best treatment involves attention to the stress factors as well as to medication. The doctor and the specialist are well able to stabilise the medical condition, usually by the continuous use of 'ventilating' drugs which prevent an attack. Additional help should only be needed if there is a cold or chest infection which exacerbates the condition. The stress factors, however, need careful attention. First, improve the mechanical ability of the lungs by breathing exercises (see Chapter 8) and practise, in particular, the calming breathing for a time when irritation may seem to be rising. The atmosphere should be kept as calm as possible and free from tensions. Any pressure, such as that of overload or time-pressures, should be kept to a minimum. Asthmatics should keep a diary with breathing spaces in it during each day and learn to say 'no' to over-commitment. Keep down all sudden movements which will push the pressure up in the lungs. Exercise gently, beginning by warming up (see Chapter 11) and do not go in for sudden bouts of gardening until wholly fit again. Being chilled, going out in a biting wind and getting over-fatigued can all make for breathing difficulties. Complementary medicine has been able to help bronchial asthma and if yours is not becoming easily stabilised on the inhalers that you use, it may be that acupuncture could be helpful. Homeopathic medicine is also used with success for bronchial asthma. Talk it over with your doctor and then contact the practitioner of your choice at the address given in Appendix 2.

Digestive difficulties

The stomach is inclined to take rather a bashing in stress. As we saw in Chapter 2, the stomach is directly affected by the stress process itself. It also reacts psychologically. The stomach lining is very susceptible to changing emotions. It becomes white when fearful, anxious or apprehensive and it becomes scarlet with rage or anger. It is not surprising, therefore, that by the end of Stage II Stress and even more so in Stage III, the stomach is giving us quite a bit of trouble. We may have any of the following problems.

A distressing symptom of stress is a 'lump in the throat' which makes eating difficult. This (if nothing abnormal has been found) is a nervous reaction. It is always worse when one has to go out for meals. It can be dealt with by means of the calming breathing technique in Chapter 8. Whenever you feel it rising, remember that *no one else knows*. Remain calm, ask for small portions only of food and take your time over eating and you will overcome it. Each occasion successfully overcome gives you encouragement for the next luncheon or dinner you have to attend.

Lump in the throat

These cover a wide range of symptoms from vague discomfort to pain and sickness. Discomfort can arise through eating or drinking too much but this occasional upset can be treated by a teaspoonful of bicarbonate of soda in a little water and a good night's sleep. If there are persistent

Indigestion and dyspepsia

feelings of nausea or of pain or actual vomitting these are signs that there are underlying problems needing medical investigation.

Heartburn
This is a burning sensation felt behind the sternum or breastbone. It is a fairly common symptom in digestive problems and in stress. It is worse at night when lying down because it is caused by a slight acid regurgitation from the stomach. If it is accompanied by the filling of the mouth with saliva (water brash) it may well be a sign of the beginnings of a peptic ulcer for which you will need help from your family doctor. With any continuing condition of indigestion or heartburn it is as well to have it investigated. If nothing wrong is found, stress has not yet caused ulceration or breached the stomach walls.

Gastritis
Gastritis is inflammation of the stomach. It can be acute, that is a sharp one-off attack which is probably not due to stress but to food poisoning, an infection such as gastric flu and occasionally it can be the result of excessive alcohol. Avoid any further irritant. Do not take aspirin. Keep warm, comfortable and drink only water, then sips of milk as the acute diarrhoea and vomiting go and the symptoms will subside in a day or two. If at the start of this attack there was swelling of the stomach (your belt has to be undone) about four hours after a meal and then diarrhoea and vomiting, call your doctor immediately as this is probably food poisoning.

Chronic gastritis
This type could well be due to stress. There is a feeling of lowness and unwellness, particularly in the morning and no appetite and there is a feeling of wanting only 'fresh' food. It is as if the stomach is unduly sensitive. Any strong smell, oil or fats, may well destroy the very delicate appetite. There is no diarrhoea or vomiting in this longer lasting but low key gastritis although there can be nausea from time to time. It is important to treat the stressed condition which is dealt with at the end of this section.

Peptic ulcer
The stomach's lining secretes mucus which protects it from all irritants and in particular from the acid necessary to break down the food into its different chemicals for use in the body. An ulcer is a breach in this wall. If it occurs in the tube leading to the stomach (the oesophagus) it is called an oesophageal ulcer, and if in the small part of the intestine,

the duodenum, it is called a duodenal ulcer. It is painful and this may be the only symptom. The timing of the pain in relation to food is usually a key to the exact place of the ulcer. For example, a gastric ulcer is irritated by food and so the pain can occur *with* eating.

A duodenal ulcer is relieved by food which neutralises the acid so hunger makes it worse, and the pain will occur *before* eating. A barium meal will clinch the diagnosis. This is a thickish and not unpleasant substance which, as it is swallowed, shows up clearly under X-ray any slight abnormality in the function of the whole of the digestive tract. If nothing abnormal is found, but you still have pain, it is due to stress which has not yet, luckily, breached the stomach wall.

Why does stress cause an ulcer?

It is a complicated mix of physiological and psychological factors acting together to make one effect. Hydrocortisone, one of the steroids, has the effect of increasing the acid secretion of the stomach, and at the same time reducing the normal output of the mucus membrane, thereby leaving the stomach wall unprotected. Anxiety, fear and anger all exacerbate the condition by raising the stress levels and thereby the steroid action. Food has the effect of neutralising the acid, so people most affected are those with stressful jobs who also go long hours with no food. These could be cab drivers, or long-distance drivers or perhaps those with shiftwork patterns which interfere with their normal appetite. It can also occur in anxious worriers and in the anger-prone who always suppress their emotions while boiling underneath. The stomach takes the brunt.

The treatment of an ulcer

If an ulcer has been found, your doctor will prescribe one of the many ulcer-healing drugs available, advise on diet and probably insist on hospitalisation to give you peace and quiet and to ensure the right medical treatment. It usually takes about six weeks to heal an ulcer. It takes much longer to deal with the stress.

Ulceration of the colon

Illness can also occur lower down in the digestive tract in the colon or bowel, and for exactly the same reasons. Oddly, there are people of a particular type of personality who are more often associated with this condition than with either gastric or duodenal ulcers. Their characteristics are excessive tidyness or meticulousness, almost to the point of neurosis. Everything must be put in a particular

227

place, and displacement causes high irritation. This is also associated with emotional dependence on one or other parent which may be transferred to a spouse. The condition of ulcerative colitis is often precipitated by the death of this supportive person, or triggered off by an attack of acute gastritis. The treatment of stress is important because this condition can relapse with stress and continue throughout life.

Irritable bowel syndrome

This is a much more common problem and (rather like pre-menstrual tension) has only recently received the acknowledgement that it exists, although people have been complaining of the symptoms for years. These symptoms are variable spells of diarrhoea and constipation, sometimes appearing together; pain in the lower abdomen with distension; and sometimes over production of gas and belching, or persistent heartburn. The difficulties with the diagnosis of this condition in the past has been the variability of the symptoms. No organism is found in the stools to account for the continuous diarrhoea, and the condition comes and goes over long periods of time. Distension of the abdomen is frequently accompanied by signs of fluid retention such as swelling of the ankles, fingers and stomach. Women often find that their rings suddenly become tight and both sexes may have extra difficulty with their waist bands. It is made very much worse by stress and it has now been recognised, and many now class it as I do, among the 'stress-induced' illnesses.

It is best treated by reducing your stress and also by increasing the fibre content of the diet. Plenty of fruit should be eaten and at least two or three vegetables a day, with the two main meals. If you have only a light lunch then it is a good plan to add fibre to breakfast in the form of bran. Eat wholemeal bread, made from stone-ground flour whenever you can get it, in preference to ordinary brown bread. Take plenty of exercise, particularly brisk walking which is best and which will help normal elimination.

The treatment of a stressed digestive system

There is no problem in healing an ulcer. One of the many antacids on the market could do the job quite well. But the ulcer will return unless you treat the stress which is the root cause.

Prevention is aimed at reducing the irritation on the sto-mach wall, as the first five points below indicate, and also at reducing the psychological effects which irritate it.

How to prevent the occurrence or recurrence of an ulcer

1   Look carefully at any drugs you may be taking, avoid all those which have salysilic acid (aspirin) in them because aspirin inflames the stomach lining and may indeed be giving you many of the symptoms that are troubling you.
2   Never drink alcohol on an empty stomach to try to give you a lift at lunchtime or after a hectic day. The stress will already have caused you pain, and alcohol inflames the stomach lining and so increases the pain. Try always to put in a lining of a glass of milk before going out for a drink or if going to a meeting or dining. It might be an idea to keep a bottle of milk in your office and have a little to line the stomach before any meeting at which you will want to drink.
3   Do not smoke on an empty stomach. Smoking is often increased during a stressful period and it actually increases the stress by increasing the rate of adrenalin production. This feels like help at the time as you are getting an extra shot of adrenalin but remember that it is raising the overall stress arousal pressure and damaging the circulation.
4   Have small, frequent meals which give the stomach a lining and reduce the stress upon it. Milk and milk foods are ideal, and also mixtures of fat and flour, eg a pasta with a light cheese sauce.
5   Change coffee drinking to milk or herb teas. Caffeine increases the adrenalin and nor adrenalin production, which increases the effect of the stress process on the stomach.

These are the psychological factors.

6   Look carefully at your life to see where the tensions are and what produces your highest emotional response. Look out, particularly, for suppressed anger and irritation. This is what is causing the damage. Read the chapter on anxiety and follow the suggestions there for dealing with your problems, particularly analysing what they are and how you react to them. Read also about the release of anger in Chapter 9. This will save your stomach. Practise the stress reduction techniques in Chapter 8, particularly the calming breathing, and use it whenever you feel irritation rising, thus stopping it at source.

229

7 The medical treatment is often long and tedious and if you feel more stressed through the inability to control a condition like irritable bowel syndrome, which is so distressing, do try homeopathic remedies. They have a high record of success with stomach and bowel problems. You will find an address to write to in Appendix 2. Talk it over with your doctor and keep him informed of progress as this may well help other patients.

Heart conditions

High blood pressure (hypertension)

Hypertension, at its simplest, just means that there is a higher than normal amount of blood going through the arteries which raises the pressure above normal. 'Normal', however, is not easy to interpret. Our blood pressure varies with what we are doing. It is lower at rest and before getting up than during heavy work because then our demands are higher. It is higher in the elderly than the young, 160/90 at age 60 is all right but too high at 20 years of age, when 120/80 would be more normal. For medicals for life insurance companies, normal is accepted at about 150/90, a little high for the young and a little low for the elderly. It is a far from normal condition though, and there can be many complex reasons for hypertension which your doctor can tell you about. We are concerned with hypertension due to over-long exposure to the mineralcorticoids in the system.

Why are there two figures for blood pressure?

As the blood goes through the heart valves they contract, then relax, regulating the flow through the different chambers. The highest peak of their contraction is the systolic pressure, the lowest point is called the diastolic pressure. The stress process, by stimulating the heart to beat faster, raises the amount of blood going through the system thereby raising the systolic blood pressure. If this high pressure is kept up over long periods of time, changes can take place in the arteries which increase their resistance to the large flow of blood. If at the same time the arteries have narrowed due to the circulating fats attaching themselves to the walls, the pressure is heightened. In this state, where both heart and circulation are under pressure and in a highly strained system, heart attacks (coronary thrombosis) and strokes (cerebral thrombosis) are possible.

What do you do about it?

1 Go to you GP and ask for your blood pressure to be taken. He will probably suggest having it taken annually.

230

2 Find out if you are in Stage II or Stage III Stress (see Chapter 2). If in Stage II, begin to exercise to improve the cardiovascular system but do not start until you have read Chapter 11 because you have to start gently and keep within three quarters of the heart capacity only.

3 At the same time reduce your tension levels to bring the increased tension in the arteries down before it does any damage (see Chapter 8). If the blood pressure is already up, bring it down with the relaxator technique every morning and evening and in addition use the mental tranquilliser in Chapter 14.

What about salt, butter and eggs?

The reason why your doctor suggests cutting down on salt, for example, is that in hypertension there is an increased salt content in the arteries. However, it is far better to control the stress response because ACTH (The hormone which in stress releases steroids from the adrenals) is responsible for our salt maintenance balance. The steroid is 18 Hydroxy Doc which is almost entirely under the control of ACTH. It is not quite as simple as it sounds – none of the chemical interactions are – but if we can keep the stress arousal levels down ACTH will not be instrumental in raising the salt levels. The same kind of situation arises with cholesterol. Cholesterol levels are high in hypertension. It is released fast into the system in high stress arousal by the action of the glucocorticoids, and kept high as long as the stress response is on. So it is vital to keep the stress levels down. At the same time if your blood pressure is already high it is advisable not to add to the problem by taking in extra salt, butter and eggs until you have got it down to near normal.

If we can control hypertension by keeping an eye on the blood pressure (there are often no symptoms that it might be high) and bringing the tension levels down, then we can go a long way towards preventing heart disease.

Many complementary techniques can help with hypertension, in particular herbal medicine and homeopathy. Acupuncture also has a record of success. Acupuncture may well be the quickest route to knowing what is going to work best for you.

How to prevent recurrence of a heart attack

If you have had a heart attack already you can prevent a recurrence. Immediately afterwards do not put any extra strain on the heart and circulation.

1   Keep warm so that the heart does not have to do it for you.

2   Avoid all high excitement, fear, anger and worry in order to keep lipids (fats and cholesterol) down.

3   Have light, not heavy meals, and rest afterwards for half an hour at least to give the circulation time to deal with digestion before exercising.

4   Cut down your weight to normal. (See table on page 141.)

5   Think about stopping smoking. Nicotine raises the adrenalin and nor adrenalin levels. This may feel good at the time, but it raises the tension in the arteries and circulation.

6   Plan to exercise starting very gradually to get your heart and circulation really fit again. Read Chapter 11 on activity.

7   Practise the tension reducing techniques in Chapter 8. If you are at all anxious about a self-monitoring programme of exercise it is a good idea to join a gymnasium with a fully qualified staff and a consultant cardiologist as its adviser. Your heart and lung function tests will be taken and you will have a carefully designed programme worked out for you which will gradually improve your heart, lungs and circulation.

8   Take your personality test (Chapter 6) and follow the stress reduction techniques for your particular type.

9   Chapter 14 will help in handling anxiety which raises tension levels.

With this lifestyle you need never have another heart attack. Chapter 10 will help you to ensure this.

Skin and joint disorders

Atopic eczema   There is a condition known as contact eczema in which a specific irritant such as a soap powder or detergent results in a skin eruption. A 24-hour patch test will identify the irritant and the only subsequent treatment is to avoid it. However, there is another cause for the eczema called 'atopic'. This is a mixture of an hereditary tendency to develop an allergy together with stress. It often occurs in childhood to those with parents who already have allergic conditions such as asthma, hay fever or urticaria. They often develop these allergies if under stress and often have persistent patches of eczema in the flexes of knees and elbows.

Several remedies are available to treat the condition medically. Often a mixture of a local steroid with an antibiotic to prevent secondary infection is useful. It is important to treat the underlying anxiety as well. Often the parents unwittingly make the situation worse by their own anxiety. They fuss about the eczema, attempt to cover it up and so make the child over conscious of it and anxious. This inevitably worsens the condition. The way to help the child is to accentuate anything he or she is good at and praise that, thereby encouraging the growth of the self-concept and of pride in achievement. Lower the significance of the eczema by taking the view that it is only slight and proof only of a sensitive skin. Children who can joke about it – 'I have a skin which is sensitive to light' – do very well indeed and the condition then clears up with age. Conversely, children whose mothers go to extraordinary lengths to cover it up or say (in front of the child) how embarrassing it is and how sensitive the child is about it, will not get rid of it easily. And this attitude will have the added effect of making the child into a morbid self-pitier, quiet and withdrawn. This kind of attitude does untold harm to the developing personality and often leads to the development of other stress-related allergies such as hay fever or asthma later on.

Treatment

These are itchy weals commonly called nettle rash or hives. They occur in very skin-sensitive people after some accident or injury and in a very stressful period after such a minor incident as an insect bite or sting. Antihistamine may help but often simple calamine lotion combined with a calm, relaxed approach will work. The main thing is not to take it seriously. Dab on some calomine lotion and get on with living and it will go all the faster.

Urticaria

This is another stress-related skin disease which can develop after a trauma such as an acute infection or, sometimes, pregnancy. There is often a family history of allergic illness and often psoriasis itself. There are no symptoms except the rash which is red and shiny with silvery scales on top. Often the scalp is involved but it can occur anywhere on the body.

Psoriasis

Like eczema and urticaria, it is not infectious or contagious and this must be made clear to everyone – family and school friends alike – and an off-hand openness about these skin conditions is an essential way of handling them to

233

forestall any social embarrassment. In the chronic stages, a stimulating treatment such as Chrysarobin is often used, and at the acute stages a soothing lotion such as camomile with Icthammol.

Treating the stress

This is the most important part of the treatment because psoriasis is usually there for life, and you have to live above it and make your own personality a winner over it. Read Chapter 15 on pampering yourself and developing your ego.

A helpful way of life is to have plenty of fresh air and sunlight, but more important is the leading of a socially outgoing life from the very beginning. Many highly successful socialites have this condition which is not noticed at all due to their out-going personalities. Learn to handle the stress, tackle any underlying anxiety and raise your resistance to stress.

The skin diseases are not suitable for acupuncture techniques but both homeopathic and herbal remedies have been found helpful. The addresses will be found in Appendix 2.

Remember the truism that other people *never notice* that you have a large nose, sticking out ears, *and psoriasis* unless you tell them. With the personality you are about to develop, no one will give your eczema, urticaria or psoriasis a second thought.

You can also dismiss it because you are behind it. You do not even see it so go ahead, live your life to the full and forget your sensitive skin in favour of your sensational personality.

Rheumatoid arthritis

This is the most common of the rheumatic diseases affecting the joints. It is a disease of the temperate zones, rather like the common cold because it does not exist in the tropics nor in the cold zones. For example, neither negroes nor eskimos suffer from the disease. Also, it is interesting to note that when arthritics visit the tropics their symptoms disappear. Women are more prone to the disease than men, being three times more likely to be affected, and the age of onset varies from 25 to 55 years of age.

The cause of rheumatoid arthritis

The reasons for the pain and swelling are that the membrane (the synovial membrane) lining the joints becomes inflamed, fluid collects between the membrane and the ends of the bones adding to the pain by pressure and the

234

joint becomes swollen and painful. Use of the joint becomes difficult through pain and stiffness.

The actual cause of these changes is obscure, but there is evidence that the condition is triggered by stress. In one study all the patients had had very stressful experiences within the three months before the onset of the disease.

There is also the well-known fact that the immune responses of the body are disturbed by the complex biochemical activity demanded by high stress arousal. In rhematoid arthritis it is the inflammatory reactions themselves of the defence system that cause the inflammation and destruction of the joints.

It is essential, therefore, as in all of these stress-induced and stress-related illnesses, to treat the stress as well as the medical condition which the stress has given rise to.

For some weeks before the actual joint damage there is indication that all is not well in the body. There is tiredness and malaise (a feeling of just not being well), loss of weight, a faster heart beat (tachicardia) and tenderness in the limbs. Another sign is sweating of the hands and of the soles of the feet.

If you feel ill, tired or are losing weight, it is a major indication that the body is fighting a battle which it may lose without help. Take notice of it, take a few days off, go to bed, keep warm, and have a good nourishing light diet and sleep as much as possible, and give the body a chance to win the battle. If rheumatoid arthritis did win you would have to do the same anyway. So do it sooner before you lose the use of your joints and have to go off work for very much longer. Chiropractors and osteopaths have both had success in treating rheumatoid arthritis and as one essential is keeping movement going the first of the complementary medicines to try might well be osteopathy. Contact the address given in Appendix 2.

Treat the stress

Long-term conflicts, particularly of a deep emotional nature, can play havoc with an immune system and it is important to resolve these as well as to find relief for the painful joints.

Do think about what disturbs your peace of mind. Doing the exercise in Chapter 14 will help, as will also practising the stress reduction techniques in Chapter 8.

Keep calm, relaxed and warm. Have a good, variable diet (see Chapter 12) with added vitamin B complex and vitamin C, take plenty of rest and be sure to keep movement going in the affected joints.

235

Significant stress component

Diabetes mellitus

Small specialist cells, the 'Islets of Langerhans', in the pancreas (near the stomach) make insulin. This turns all the sugars in our food into glucose, a substance which can be used by the body for energy. If these cells fail or produce very little or poor insulin the sugar not used up circulates freely in the bloodstream. The body attempts to dilute it, and thirst is usually the first sign of diabetes.

It is a disease of the mechanised, industrial countries who overload themselves with sugar and junk food. There is only 0.1 per cent in the population of primitive countries and 7 per cent in the industrial West. Twenty per cent of cases in the UK are among the young and the cause is mainly hereditary. Eighty per cent, however, is of late origin occurring in the obese, over 50s. This type often follows a physical injury, illness or accident or some emotional stress to the system. It is thought that the anxiety and emotional distress affects the pituitary adrenal system which in turn affects the cells causing a reduction in the amount of insulin. As stress is implicated it has to be treated as well as the medical condition.

Stress is also caused by the diagnosis itself. However, diabetics can lead full, active lives. Indeed, some of our top sportsmen have been diabetics. Often people are scared of diabetic coma. It is true that drowsiness can occur if you have had all of your insulin for the day and you are late with lunch. Always carry two sugar lumps or two biscuits to eat if you are likely to be late with a meal and this will carry you over without difficulty. The British Diabetic Association (the address is in Appendix 2) will help with all the information you need about the condition. Contact also Healthline as they have tapes on diabetes. Then, reassured that you can lead a normal life, plan to reduce your anxiety and tensions with Part II. If you feel you need help with talking over and handling your problems get in touch with the British Assocation of Counselling to find out your nearest counsellor. They are countrywide now so you should have no difficulty in finding one near you. Homeopathic medicine has had success in reversing the course of diabetes, so it is well worthwhile contacting a practitioner and taking his treatment.

Cancer

What do we know and believe about cancer? It is important to get at the truth because cancer is one of the illnesses

236

which is often curable in its early stages and there are now many tests which make this early detection and cure possible.

People who go for these check-ups see themselves as intelligent, responsible, well-organised and healthy; whereas those who do not, see those who do as worriers, scared and nervous and hypochondriacs. We obviously have to change some attitudes. It is intelligent to go and take advantage of check-ups or screening techniques at least once a year and to know the early signs of any major trouble in order to nip it in the bud. This is not being a hypochondriac – it is taking a healthy responsibility for your own health and well-being.

Breast cancer

Only a minority of women who were asked in a recent survey knew that 85 per cent of breast cancer, if detected early, can be cured. Only 15 per cent of lumps in the breast are malignant and these lumps can be felt very easily by self examination of the breasts. It is well worth doing for the sake of a few extra minutes. If you do feel a lump go straight to your doctor who will make arrangements for it to be shelled out. This is done through a small nick in the skin which is unlikely to be seen when it heals.

Uterine cancer

Most women in that survey had heard of the test for cervical cancer but did not know that there is also a test for uterine cancer. It is well worthwhile having these tests before there is evidence of cancer.

Lung cancer

This is shown up on an X-ray of the lungs which is a simple precaution to take, particularly if you are a smoker. Lung cancer is not among those which are easily curable by the time one is aware of the symptoms, so it is well worthwhile taking the precaution of an annual X-ray.

Colonic and rectal cancer

These are now the most prevalent forms of cancer. There is a test for this, and a do-it-yourself guaiac test in which you can take small samples of your stools three mornings running. You put them on glass slides (provided) and send these, through your doctor, to the public health laboratory which will test for blood in the stool which may point to the need to go to your doctor for a full rectal examination.

What is probably needed above all is a clear knowledge of the warning signs of cancer. These are:

237

1   A lump or thickening in the breast.
2   Any unusual bleeding or discharge from any orifice.
3   Any change in a wart or a mole, ie bleeding or sudden growth.
4   Any sore which does not heal.
5   Any persistent cough or continuing hoarseness.
6   Any change in bowel or bladder habits (not just the odd day, but a definite change over weeks).
7   Persistent indigestion or difficulty in swallowing.

All of these are signs that there is something not quite right with the functioning of the body and although they may not indicate cancer, something is going wrong and whatever it is should be investigated so as to catch it in the early stages while it can still be cured. Do not wait until things become serious.

If you do find that you have cancer of any part of the body do not accept this as the end of your world. People who make quite dramatic recoveries from serious illness have several points in common:

A refusal to give in to the condition.
A definite and serious intention to get themselves cured.
Fixing on a definite goal or project to live for.
Taking the trouble to find a doctor or specialist who is as positive as they themselves are.

The two main things are the refusal to give in and fixing on a definite future goal to work towards. Even cancer which has been left quite late and has become serious, has been vanquished by the determination to win through which in turn has mobilised and strengthened the body's own healing processes.

I have not gone into the relationship between stress and cancer because it is only at the supposition stage although there is now developing a body of evidence for it. What is important is the calming of the tension, anxieties and fears of the condition itself. It is curable in the early stages and even people who have been told they have a terminal condition have been cured through their own common-sense approach to it, together with their determination to support their body's fight against it. Do not accept that something is incurable. The body is wiser than we know.

For help and advice, if you or someone in your family has cancer, get in touch with the Bristol Cancer Help Centre. (See Appendix 2.)

Penny Brohn, who helped to start the centre, had cancer herself and she said that the moment she was told she had cancer she changed and became a bundle of fear and terror and was convinced she was going to die, until sanity returned and she realised that the *word* cancer itself had caused all this – not the illness. As soon as she came to terms with the word, her cure was under way. Through this experience she is able to help others to realise that cancer is only a word. The illness is only an illness like any other one that the body's immune and defence systems deal with and conquer every day. Your system can conquer it too.

CHAPTER 18

You are not alone

In this final chapter I want to take you back to Chapter 10, the chapter on lifestyle. You remember that there I said that we were all destined to be so much greater, so much healthier, so much happier than most of us are today. This is true from what we know of our genetic potential. Not one of us succeeds in reaching even a quarter of our potential. We have powers, power of the mind, the power of thought and the power of vision which few of us in the industrialised Western world have tapped. We have not the time to stop and think, let alone the time to be quiet and develop the powers within us.

Stillness

Being still, having the time to think our thoughts and let the mind play over new ideas and demonstrate its powers is a talent we have lost. As a child, the one thing I remember about visits to my great-grandparents was the peace and the stillness of the evenings which nothing ever disturbed. The log fire burned, the lamps were lit and the room seemed bathed in a warm glow. My great-grandparents were great readers and my chief memory is of sitting on a big, soft, squashy leather hassock looking at firelight, weaving my own stories. There was a stillness and calmness about those two figures content with their books. They would smile warmly and nod to me if I caught their eye and back they would go to their reading. It was a companionable quiet in which everyone was content and no one made any demands upon another. Today, by contrast, there are too many demands made upon us and there is no time to be ourselves. But there is help out there in our community.

You have pastoral care

One of the places where we can be quiet with our thoughts and be our own person is in our faith, whatever it is. Much of the appeal of the Eastern mythologies and religions at present is in the peace that they engender through their meditation techniques. Yet, we all have the ability to still

240

the mind and to be at peace; it is inherent in every one of us. In Christian teachings we have meditation and contemplation. They are one of the oldest parts of our religion together with the laying on of hands at the healing services. We hear little about them, but they are there, and they are there for us. If you are interested in Christian meditation ask your priest or vicar if he would have a weekly group for prayer and meditation. Some people find it a great solace, giving them renewed strength and courage to face the rest of the week. In some groups there is a coming together or exploration of the differences in oriental meditation and the Christian approach. If you would like to further this in your group there are books on the subject. (See Appendix 1).

We are living at a very interesting and exciting time for health care when different trends seem to be coming together for the benefit of our health. We have Church leaders exploring other religions to see what they have to offer and recommending that some religious communities might well explore forms of Eastern meditation and, in fact, this is now being done. *An exciting time to live*

There is the beginning of the coming together of orthodox medicine with complementary medicine as seen in the setting up of the British Holistic Medical Association, a trend we mentioned in Chapter 16. This association is now developing an associate membership for the practitioners of complementary medicine. This is a big step forward for a medical association.

So we have East meeting West in both religious practice and in medicine, or at very least the start of the dialogue between them. This can only work to our advantage, so the future is full of promise for a more holistic approach to care. In addition, the public now has its own college for health.

The College for Health aims to do for us, the patients, what the Royal College of Physicians, Surgeons, or General Practitioners does for doctors. It aims to look after our interests, to further our education in health matters by putting on courses, meetings and seminars to give information on the use of the health services. For example, they give information on how to go about getting a second opinion if you need one. It has already developed Healthline, through which, for the price of a telephone call, you can listen to tapes of your choice on different illnesses. *You have a college*

241

These give an outline of the symptoms and treatment, give advice on when to see your doctor, and finally give a list of helpful self-help groups for that particular condition. These recorded tapes are from two to six minutes long and already cover 30 or more subjects. You can suggest topics you would like to see covered. The college aims to be an influential pressure group to press for better health care for its members. For example, there is a members' lobby which will take your particular problems right to the top. They also put out a magazine for members called *Self Health* which gives un-biassed information on various topics and remedies, uninfluenced by advertising pressure. It carries no advertisements whatsoever, a welcome innovation among the myriads of health magazines on sale today.

You have information on 1300 organisations for health

Another interesting innovation is the setting up of the Institute of Complementary Medicine. They now have directories of registered practitioners in many of the complementary therapies, in particular the five major therapies dealt with in Chapter 16: acupuncture, homeopathy, medical herbalism, osteopathy and chiropractics. In addition, they have an information service containing details of some 1300 organisations around the country which deal with preventive medicine and self-help groups. They are setting up public information points which they call PIPS where the public can get help and advice. (See Appendix 2) They have 57 at present, all manned by volunteers.

You are not alone in wanting to become fit and energetic

Everyone of us wants to shed those odd symptoms of stress which we all have from time to time. The tension headache, the dyspeptic stomach, the odd pain in the joints, the feeling that you just want to sleep for a week.

We all want to be healthier; we all intend to get up early and go for that early morning run. We know that we will feel better after it. We all intend to slim down; to lose that stomach and the tyre around the waist. We intend to give up chocolate, cakes and sugar – tomorrow. Today we feel stressed and deprived. The whole difficulty is doing it alone because it takes energy and effort and willpower and all of those things we have not got if we have only just got over a stress illness.

But you are not alone. There is a great deal of help out there in the community just waiting to be tapped. But perhaps we would like something, some support from a group right here in the community, in our own community? Well why not. The solution is easy why not form your own? I started a Phoenix Group in 1982 and there is nothing easier than getting a group together. A little piece in your parish magazine or in the local paper would interest an editor into putting it in free for you because the forming of a group to come together on one evening a week, in order to solve problems and develop a lifestyle which is less stressful, and to learn and practice stress reduction techniques, is news. Ask him to insert your telephone number and give the date and address of the first meeting. You will be surprised at the response because nearly everyone of us thinks that we are under stress. It is a good plan to start it in the kitchen where there is coffee ready and let everyone help themselves and carry a cup through to the meeting. This gets over the first hurdle. Then let everyone introduce themselves saying who they are, what they hope to achieve from the meeting and what they are able to give. You may have doctors, social workers, teachers, nurses or housewives who had studied Yoga; all are able to bring their own expertise to the group. If you are interested in developing this idea you could join the Stress Foundation which aims to educate and inform on all aspects of stress and its control. The Foundation develops training courses for industry, publishes information leaflets, pamphlets, holds conferences and has a pamphlet on *How To Organise Phoenix Groups*. (See Appendix 2)

*   *   *

You are not alone, there is a lot of help out there in the community and you yourself can play a big part of the ever growing self-help movement. The reward includes having your own support group right on your doorstep.

Stress is a problem faced by every one of us at some times in our lives. Those of us who are now knowledgeable in Stressmanship are, in a way, in the very privileged position of not only being able to help ourselves, but also to help others. As you now know, stress can be a potent ally, but all too frequently in the type of lives that most of us lead, we tend to keep it on at full blast, dissipating our reserves of energy, and driving ourselves to drink, drugs, despair and destruction. It is high time to call a halt to this wasteful destruction of human life by the misuse of a power given to us for a life-saving purpose. Let us get back to a sane and healthy way of living, keeping the stress response for what it is really meant to be – a life saver, not a life destroyer.

APPENDIX 1

Further Reading

The Alternative Health Guide, Brian Inglis & Ruth West.
Michael Joseph, London, 1983.

Asserting Yourself, Dr Marsha Lineham & Dr Kelly Egan.
Century, London, 1983.

Beat Heart Disease, Dr Risteard Mulcahy. Martin Dunitz,
London, 1979.

Beating Depression, Dr John Rush. Century, London,
1983.

Broken Heart, The. J L Lynch, New York, 1977.

Eating and Allergy. Robert Eagle, London, 1979.

Fears and Phobias, Dr Tony Whitehead. Sheldon Press,
London, 1980.

How to Stay Well, Pauvo Airola. Phoenix, Arizona, 1974.

Living After a Stroke, Diana Law & Barbara Paterson.
Souvenir Press, London, 1980.

Loneliness. Why It Happens and How To Overcome It, Dr
Tony Lake. Sheldon Press, London, 1981.

Man Adapting, Rene Dubos. Yale University Press, 1985.

Managing Anxiety & Stress, James Archer Jr. A.D.,
Indiana, 1982.

Meeting Schools of Oriental Meditation, Herbert Slade.
Lutterworth Educational, 1973.

Overcoming Arthritis, Dr Frank Dudley. Audrey Hart, 1981.

Relaxation Response, The, Herbert Benson. William Morrow, New York, 1975.

Stress & The Art Of Biofeedback, Barbara S Brown. Harper & Row, New York, 1977.

Stress Strategies, C B Scrignar. Karger, 1983.

APPENDIX 2

Helpful Addresses

Acupuncture	British Medical Acupuncture Society 67/69 Chancery Lane, London WC2 1AF. For doctors skilled in acupuncture. Register of British Acupuncturists 34 Alderney Street, London, SW1V 3EU. This covers the non-medical societies.
Alcohol problems	ACCEPT (Alcoholism Community Centres for Education, Prevention and Treatment) Western Hospital, Seagrave Road, London SW6 1RZ. Tel: 01 381 3155. National Council on Alcoholism 3 Grosvenor Crescent, London SW1X 7EE. Tel: 01 235 4182. For advice on alcohol information centres and where to seek help.
Arthritis	British Rheumatism & Arthritis Association 6 Grosvenor Crescent, London, SW1.
Asthma	Asthma Research Council 12 Penbridge Square, London W2 4EH. Tel: 01 229 1149
Cancer	Bristol Cancer Help Centre Grove House, Cornwallis Grove, Clifton, Bristol BS8 4PG
Chiropractors	British Chiropractors Association 5 First Avenue, Chelmsford, Essex CM1 1RX

Complementary medicine	Institute of Complementary Medicine 21 Portland Place, London W1N 3AF. Tel: 01 636 9543
Counselling	British Association for Counselling 1a Little Church Street, Rugby, Warwickshire. Tel: (0788) 78328
	Westminster Pastoral Foundation 23 Kensington Square, London W8 5HN. Tel: 01 937 6956. Counselling for individuals, family and marital problems.
Diabetes	British Diabetic Association, The 10 Queen Anne Street, London W1M 0BD. Tel: 01 323 1531 Will give help and advice on local branches.
Depression	Depressives Associated 19 Merley Ways, Wimborne Minster, Dorset BH21 1QN. Tel: 0202 883957 A national association of self-help groups. Telephone for information about your nearest.
Drug abuse	Standing Conference of Drug Abuse 3 Blackburn Road, London NW6 1XA. Tel: 01 328 6556. For advice on organisations dealing with drug misuse, and information on sources of counselling.
Family	Family Network (National Childrens Home) 85 Highbury Park, London N5. Tel: 01 224 2033. Phone-in help service for families in distress.
	Women's Aid Federation 374 Grays Inn Road, London WC1. Tel: 01 837 9316. Advice on refuges for battered women.

OPUS (Organisations for Parents under Stress)
29 Newmarket Way, Hornchurch, Essex RM12 6DR. Tel: 04024 51538.
Help for parents and advice on how to find a local group.

Healthline
PO Box 499, London E2 9PU.

Herbal
medicine

National Institute of Herbal Medicine
148 Forest Road, Tunbridge Wells, Kent. Tel: 0892 30400.

Holistic
medicine

British Medical Holistic Association
179 Gloucester Place, London NW1 6DX. Tel: 01 262 5299.
Association for doctors interested on the holistic approach.

Homeopathy

Information Service, Homeopathic Development Foundation Ltd
19a Cavendish Square, London W1M 9AD. Tel: 01 629 3204.

Migraine

Migraine Trust, The
45 Great Ormonde Street, London WC1N 3HD. Tel: 01 287 2676.
Gives advice over the telephone.

City of London Migraine Clinic
22 Charterhouse Square, London, EC1.
Tel: 01 251 3322.

Princess Margaret Migraine Clinic
Charing Cross Hospital, Fulham Palace Road, London W6 8RF.
Tel: 01 741 7833.
Both the above clinics will treat attacks on a casualty basis. At other times, ask to be referred by your GP.

Naturopathy

British Neuropathic and Osteopathic Association
Frazer House, 6 Netherhall Gardens, London NW3. Tel: 01 435 8728.

	Runs clinics and the British College of Naturopathy and Osteopathy which provides a four-year course in both subjects. Publishes a list of its practitioners.
Osteopathy	Register of Osteopaths 1–4 Suffolk Street, London SW1. Tel: 01 839 2060. List of practitioners in the UK.
Phobias	Open Door Association, The 447 Pensby Road, Heswall, Wirrall, Merseyside L61 9PG. (for agorophobics) Phoebic Society, The 4 Cheltenham Road, Chormon-Cumhardy, Manchester M21 1QN. Tel: 061 881 1937. (all phobias)
Psychotherapists	The British Association of Psychotherapists 121 Hendon Lane, London N3 3PR. Tel: 01 346 1747.
Skin problems	National Eczema Society Tavistock House North, Tavistock Square, London WC1H 9SR. Tel: 01 388 4097. Information about the problem and its management. Psoriasis Association, The 7 Milton Street, Northampton NN2 7JG. Tel: 0604 711129.
Smoking	ASH (Action on Smoking and Health) Margaret Pyke House, 27–35 Mortimer Street, London W1N 7RJ. Tel: 01 637 9843.
Stress	Stress Foundation, The Cedar House, Yalding, Kent ME18 6JD. Tel: 0622 814431. (Leaflets and publications on aspects of stress).

Suicide   Samaritans, The
                 Listed in every local telephone directory.
                 A telephone service for those at the end
                 of their tether and contemplating suicide.

Yoga   British Wheel of Yoga
                 80 Lechampton Road, Cheltenham,
                 Gloucestershire.
                 Lists all the qualified teachers of Yoga.

Index

Learning
Resource Centre
Stockton
Riverside College